Contents

Osteoporosis
Osteoporosis

Stuart H. Ralston
Professor of Medicine and Bone Metabolism,
University of Aberdeen Medical School,
Aberdeen, UK.

Michael Kleerekoper
Professor of Medicine,
Department of Internal Medicine,
Wayne State University,
Detroit, Michigan, USA.

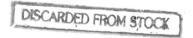

MOSBY
An imprint of Elsevier Science Limited.

© 2002 Elsevier Science Limited.

The Publisher's policy is to use **paper manufactured from sustainable forests**

M Mosby is a registered trademark of Elsevier Science Limited.

ISBN 0-7234-3324-0

Cataloguing in Publication Data
Catalogue records for this book are available from the US Library of Congress and the British Library.

Note
Medical knowledge is constantly changing. As new information becomes available, changes in treatment, procedures, equipment and the use of drugs become necessary. The editors/authors/contributors and the publishers have taken care to ensure that the information given in this text is accurate and up to date. However, readers are strongly advised to confirm that the information, especially with regard to drug usage, complies with the latest legislation and standards of practice.

Printed by Grafos S.A. Arte sobre papel, Spain.

04834022

Abbreviations

BMD	bone mineral density
BMP	bone morphogenic protein
BUA	broadband ultrasound attenuation
ESR	erythrocyte sedimentation rate
DEXA	dual energy X-ray absorptiometry
ER	oestrogen receptor
HRT	hormone replacement therapy
LRP	lipoprotein receptor-related protein
OI	osteogenesis imperfecta
OPG	osteoprotegerin
PTH	parathyroid hormone
QCT	quantitative computed tomography
QUS	quantitative ultrasound
RANK	receptor activator of nuclear factor kappa B
RANKL	RANK ligand
SERM	selective oestrogen receptor modulator
SOS	speed of sound
SOST	sclerostin
TGF	transforming growth factor
VDR	vitamin D receptor

Introduction

Osteoporosis is one of the most important public health problems in developed societies, and an emerging problem of increasing clinical and economic significance in developing countries.[1] It is a common disease predominantly affecting older people, which is characterized by reduced bone mass, microarchitectural deterioration of bone tissue and an increased risk of fragility fractures. These fractures affect about 30% of women and 12% of men at some point during life, accounting for treatment costs of £1.4 billion in the UK and $18 billion in the USA. Most general practitioners and primary care physicians are likely to have several hundred patients on their list with osteoporosis, although many of these patients and their doctors are unaware that they have the condition. This is because osteoporosis does not cause symptoms until a fragility fracture occurs, and even then, the fracture may not be recognized as a complication of osteoporosis. Awareness of osteoporosis has now become a key issue in clinical practice, however, because of the ease with which the diagnosis can be made using bone densitometry and because of the availability of effective agents for prevention and treatment.

Definition and Epidemiology

Osteoporosis is defined to exist when bone mineral density (BMD) values fall more than 2.5 standard deviations (T-score units) below the population average in young healthy adults.[2] Patients with lesser reductions in bone mass are classified as having osteopaenia, which is defined to exist when BMD T-score values fall to between −1 and −2.5. Osteoporosis does not cause symptoms, and is therefore clinically silent until a fracture occurs. When fractures do occur in an osteporotic patient, the diagnosis of severe or established osteoporosis is made (Table 1).

Table 1. Definition of osteoporosis	
BMD T-score value/ fracture history	**Diagnosis**
Greater than −1.0	Normal
Between −1.0 and −2.5	Osteopaenia
Below −2.5	Osteoporosis
Below −2.5 and fragility fracture	Established osteoporosis

The prevalence of osteoporosis increases with age, reflecting the fact that bone mass falls with increasing age (Figure 1). Age-related bone loss occurs in both sexes, but women suffer an accelerated phase of bone loss after the menopause because of oestrogen deficiency, which increases bone turnover and at the same time causes uncoupling of bone resorption and bone formation. The bone loss that results from postmenopausal oestrogen deficiency explains why osteoporosis is more prevalent in women. By the age of 60, approximately 15% of all women have osteoporosis, and this figure increases to 38% by the age of 80.[3]

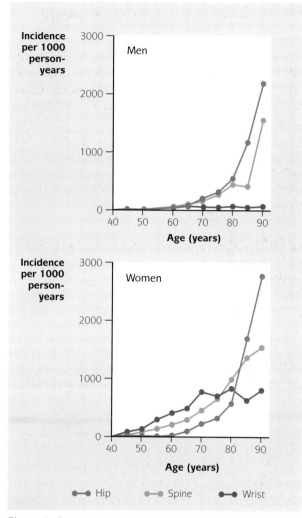

Figure 1. Changes in incidence of common osteoporotic fractures with age. Reprinted with permission Elsevier Science from Cooper C, Melton LJ. Epidemiology of osteoporosis. *Trends Endocrinol Metab* 1992; **3**: 224–229.[1]

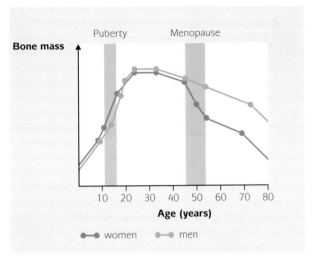

Figure 2. Changes of bone mass with age in men and women.

Osteoporosis has few physical signs and, because of this, the diagnosis is difficult to make clinically until the patient has suffered a fragility fracture. Fragility fractures are typical of osteoporosis and are defined to occur when the fracture happens spontaneously, or is triggered by a fall from standing height or less. Vertebral fractures are under-diagnosed. Whilst some present acutely with sudden back pain, others occur insidiously, causing the patient to present at an advanced stage with height loss and kyphosis. The incidence of all osteoporotic fractures increases progressively with age (Figure 1), mirroring the fact that bone mass falls with age (Figure 2). Whilst the pattern is similar in both sexes for hip and spine fractures, men are relatively protected from wrist fractures at all ages and the incidence of wrist fractures in women reaches a plateau from the age of 70. This is thought to be due to differences in the patterns of falling; men are less likely to fall on an outstretched

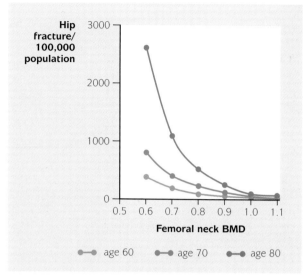

Figure 3. Effect of age and bone density on incidence of hip fracture. Reproduced with permission from Laet CE *et al*. Bone density and risk of hip fracture in men and women: cross sectional analysis. *Br Med J* 1997; **315**: 221–225.[4]

arm than women at all ages, whereas women appear to lose the protective reflex of extending their arm in the event of a fall as they get older.

Reduced bone mass contributes to the increased incidence of fractures with increasing age, but this is not the whole story. Recent studies have shown that the incidence of hip fracture greatly increases with increasing age independently of changes in bone density (Figure 3).[4] This reflects the importance of falls to the pathogenesis of fracture in the elderly due to factors such as reduced muscle strength, poor balance and loss of visual acuity.[5]

There are marked ethnic differences in the risk of osteoporotic fractures. This has been particularly well documented for hip fractures which are common in Caucasian populations, but much less common in other ethnic groups

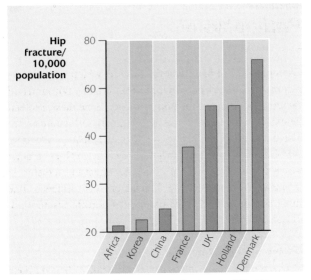

Figure 4. Prevalence of osteoporotic fracture in different ethnic groups.

such as Asians and Africans (Figure 4).[6] Several factors contribute to these differences, including lifestyle, diet and genetic determinants of bone density, as well as differences in skeletal geometry. The lower risk of hip fracture in Asians is thought to be due to a shorter hip axis length, which is biomechanically more favourable in the event of a fall.[7] Ethnic differences in bone mass also play a role and probably account for the lower incidence of fractures in African-Americans as compared with Caucasians.

Pathophysiology

Osteoporosis is a multifactorial disease, which is caused by a complex interaction between genetic and environmental factors that influence the bone turnover, bone mass, skeletal geometry and the risk of falling (Figure 5). Osteoporosis can also occur as a complication of various genetic, endocrine, metabolic and inflammatory diseases that influence bone turnover, and as a result of drugs that affect the skeleton or influence the risk of falling. The factors that influence bone mass and other determinants of osteoporotic fracture are discussed below.

Bone structure

The normal skeleton consists of cortical and trabecular bone types. About 80% of the skeleton is made of cortical bone, which forms an envelope around the outside of all bones. The remaining

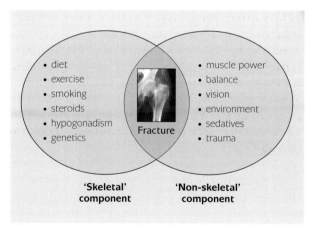

Figure 5. Role of skeletal and non-skeletal factors in the pathogenesis of fracture.

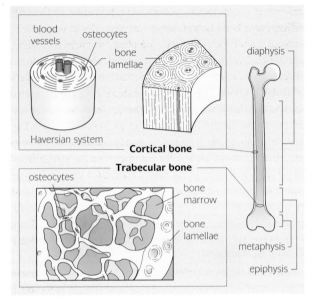

Figure 6. Bone structure.

20% is trabecular bone, which makes up the interior of the long bones and flat bones, most of the vertebral bodies and some other bones such as the calcaneus (Figure 6). Cortical bone is arranged in Haversian systems, which consist of a series of concentric lamellae of bone tissue containing osteocytes which surround a central canal that contains blood vessels. Nutrients reach the centre of the bone by an interconnecting system of narrow channels (canaliculi) that run between osteocytes and lining cells on the bone surface. Trabecular bone is much less dense than cortical bone, because marrow spaces containing blood vessels, osteoprogenitor cells and haemopoietic cells separate the individual bony trabeculae. These trabeculae contain osteocytes and canaliculi as in cortical bone, but here the bone lamellae run parallel to the bone surface, rather than concentrically.

The cells of bone

The main cells of bone are osteoblasts, osteocytes, bone lining cells and osteoclasts. Osteoblasts are cuboidal mononuclear cells which are responsible for new bone formation. Osteoblasts differentiate from bone marrow stromal cells in response to various stimuli, including bone morphogenic proteins (BMPs), parathyroid hormone (PTH), calcitriol and sex hormones (Figure 7a). Recent work has shown that the stimulatory effects of BMPs on bone formation are inhibited by a protein called sclerostin (SOST), which binds to BMPs.[8] The combined effects of the above factors stimulate the expression of two key transcription factors called CBFA1 and osterix in pre-osteoblasts. These factors bind to the regulatory regions of target genes and act to promote the coordinated changes in gene expression that are necessary for osteoblast differentiation and function.[9,10] Osteocytes are small mononuclear cells with elongated cytoplasmic processes which are derived from osteoblasts that become buried in bone matrix during bone formation. Osteocytes are thought to act as sensors of mechanical strain in the skeleton.[11] Bone lining cells are flattened cells of mesenchymal origin which cover the bone surface. The function of lining cells is incompletely understood, but recent work suggests that they are involved in "cleaning" collagenous bone matrix from the bottom of resorption lacunae and initiating bone formation.[12]

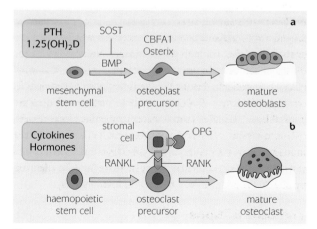

Figure 7. Regulation of osteoblast (a) and osteoclast (b) differentiation.

Osteoclasts are multinucleated cells of haemopoietic origin which are responsible for bone resorption.[13] Osteoclast differentiation is promoted by various hormones, including PTH, calcitriol and thyroid hormone, and inflammatory cytokines like interleukin-1 and tumour necrosis factor. These factors promote osteoclast differentiation and activity by stimulating production of a molecule called RANK ligand (RANKL) on osteoblasts and stromal cells. The RANKL then interacts with a receptor present on osteoclast precursors called RANK (receptor activator of nuclear factor kappa B) to promote osteoclast differentiation and function. The RANK–RANKL interaction is blocked by another molecule called osteoprotegerin (OPG), which is a "decoy" ligand for RANK and which acts a potent inhibitor of osteoclast formation. When formed, mature osteoclasts form a tight seal over the bone surface and resorb bone by secreting hydrochloric acid and proteolytic enzymes such as collagenase and cathepsin K onto the bone surface.

Bone matrix

The main organic component of bone matrix is type I collagen, which is a fibrillar protein formed from two collagen α1 and one collagen α2 chains.[14] Following translation within the osteoblast cytoplasm, the individual pro-collagen chains self assemble to form a triple helix. The collagen is then secreted into the extracellular space, where the terminal portions of the chains (pro-peptides) are removed by proteolytic digestion. The triple helical domains that remain then become linked by specialized covalent bonds (pyridinium cross-links) which stabilize the individual collagen fibrils and help to give bone its tensile strength (Figure 8).[15] Osteoblasts also secrete small amounts of other proteins, including growth factors, cytokines and other extracellular matrix proteins. These are thought to be involved in mediating the attachment of bone cells to bone matrix, and in regulating bone cell activity during the process of bone remodelling. Bone matrix undergoes mineralization about 10 days after it has been laid down by osteoblasts. This involves the deposition of calcium phosphate crystals, in the form of

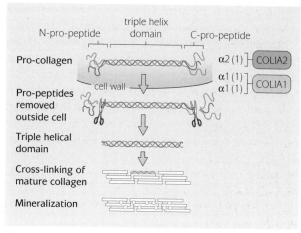

Figure 8. Type I collagen assembly and structure.

hydroxyapatite $[Ca_{10}(PO_4)_6(OH)_2]$ into the spaces between collagen fibrils. Mineralization confers upon bone the properties of hardness and mechanical rigidity, which complement the tensile strength and elasticity derived from bone matrix.

Bone remodelling

Bone remodelling is a process of renewal and repair which occurs throughout life, and is responsible for normal modelling of bones during growth and repair of damage which is sustained by the skeleton throughout life (Figure 9).[16] Bone remodelling is divided into phases of resorption: reversal, formation and quiescence. It has been estimated that, at any one time, approximately 90% of bone surface in the adult skeleton is in the quiescent phase and the remaining 10% is undergoing active remodelling. Bone remodelling commences with attraction of osteoclasts to the site that is to be resorbed. The mechanisms which determine where and when resorption occurs are poorly understood, but may involve release of osteoclast-chemotactic factors from areas of skeletal microdamage. After osteoclasts have removed a certain amount of bone, they undergo programmed cell death and disappear from the resorption lacunae, in the reversal phase.

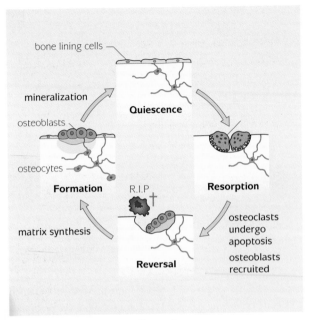

Figure 9. The bone remodelling cycle.

Osteoblast precursors are then attracted into the resorption cavity and begin to lay down new bone matrix, within the previously excavated resorption lacuna. The newly formed matrix (osteoid) then becomes mineralized to produce mature bone, which restores the remodelling site to a quiescent state.

Whatever the underlying cause, osteoporosis occurs because there is an imbalance between the amount of bone which is gained during bone remodelling as the result of growth and development and the amount of bone which is lost because of remodelling as the result of age, sex hormone deficiency, drugs and disease states (Figure 10).

Regulation of peak bone mass and bone loss

Bone mass increases steadily during childhood and adolescence to reach a peak between the ages of 25 and 35 (Figure 2). Peak bone mass is reached slightly earlier in women

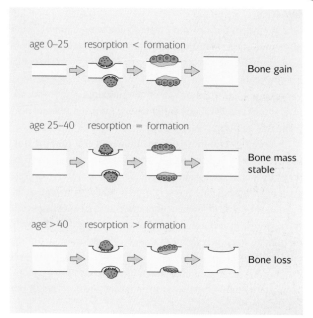

Figure 10. Scenarios for bone gain and bone loss.

due to their earlier pubertal development, although the absolute amount of bone mass achieved is greater in men due to their greater body size. There is a gradual fall in bone mass after the age of about 40 in both sexes, due to the fact that bone resorption tends to slightly exceed bone formation in each bone remodelling cycle. In women, however, there is a phase of accelerated bone loss around the age of 50, due to the effects of oestrogen deficiency after the menopause. Oestrogen normally suppresses bone turnover in the adult and its deficiency results in increased bone turnover with partial "uncoupling" of bone resorption from bone formation, such that a small amount of bone is lost with each remodelling cycle. The rate of bone loss tends to slow down between the ages of 60 and 70, but there is a tendency for it to increase once again in the elderly, possibly because of reduced physical activity. Several factors contribute to the regulation of bone mass and bone loss, and these are discussed in more detail below.

Genetics

Genetic factors play an important role in the regulation of bone mass and other phenotypes relevant to the pathogenesis of osteoporosis.[17] Twin and family studies have shown that genetic factors account for between 70% and 85% of individual variance in bone mass and other determinants of osteoporotic fracture risk, such as body weight, bone turnover, femoral neck geometry and ultrasound properties of bone (Table 2).

In keeping with these observations, several investigators have reported that a family history of hip fracture predicts the development of fracture independently of bone mass.[20] Current evidence suggests that many different genes contribute to the regulation of bone mass and other determinants of osteoporotic fracture risk in normal individuals, but so far, only a few of these have been identified (Table 3). Polymorphisms in the vitamin D receptor, oestrogen receptor α, collagen type I α1

Table 2. Heritability of phenotypes relevant to osteoporosis[18,19]	
Phenotype	**Heritability***
Bone density	
Spine BMD	0.78 (0.28–1.28)
Femoral neck BMD	0.84 (0.30–1.38)
Wrist BMD	0.46 (0.02–0.90)
Quantitative ultrasound/skeletal geometry	
BUA	0.53 (0.05–1.01)
SOS	0.61 (0.14–1.08)
Hip axis length	0.62 (0.22–1.02)
Bone turnover	
Serum bone-specific alkaline phosphatase	0.77 (0.70–0.82)
Urine DPD	0.59 (0.53–0.64)
Serum PTH	0.63 (0.57–0.68)
* mean (95% confidence interval)	

gene and transforming growth factor β gene have been shown to play a role in regulation of BMD, although the contribution of individual genes is modest (between 1% and 2%). Less commonly, mutations in a single gene can have major effects on bone mass. The classic example of this is osteogenesis

Table 3. Genes associated with osteoporosis

Gene	Allelic variants	Role in bone metabolism
Vitamin D receptor[22]	Involved in calcium absorption and bone cell differentiation	Several polymorphisms identified which may affect mRNA stability and receptor function. Effects on bone mass may depend on calcium intake
Oestrogen receptor[23]	Mediates effect of oestrogen on bone	Intronic and promoter polymorphisms associated with small effects on BMD, by mechanisms which are unclear. Rare inactivating mutations described which disrupt receptor function
Aromatase[24]	Converts androgens to oestrogen in target tissues	Rare inactivating mutations disrupt enzyme function, leading to severe osteoporosis
COLIA1[25]	Collagen is the major protein of bone. α I chain, encoded by COLIA1 genes	Mutations affecting coding regions of COLIA1 and COLIA2 cause osteogenesis imperfecta due to production of abnormal collagen, or reduced amounts of collagen. Polymorphism in regulatory region of COLIA1 associated with reduced bone mass and increased bone fragility by altering normal ratio of COLIA1/COLIA2

Table 3. Continued

Gene	Allelic variants	Role in bone metabolism
Transforming growth factor (TGF) β1[26,27]	Involved in regulating osteoclast and osteoblast activity	Mutations affect binding of mature TGF β to the inhibitory LAP subunit of TGF β, leading to Engelmann's disease, characterized by osteosclerosis of long bones. Various common polymorphisms described which are associated with bone mass
LRP5[21,28]	Involved in regulation of bone formation	Inactivating (recessive) mutations cause osteoporosis–pseudoglioma syndrome. Activating (dominant) mutations cause high bone mass

imperfecta, which is most often caused by mutations in the collagen type I α1 and type I α2 genes. These mutations result in the production of abnormal, or reduced, amounts of type I collagen, causing reduced bone mass and increased bone fragility. Severe osteoporosis also occurs in patients with inactivating mutations of the oestrogen gene and the aromatase gene, both of which are required for the actions of oestrogens on bone. Inactivating mutations of lipoprotein receptor-related protein-5 (LRP5) gene cause the osteoporosis–pseudoglioma syndrome.[21] Osteoporosis occurs in this condition because LRP5 plays a key role in regulating bone formation during skeletal development.

Sex hormones
Oestrogen and testosterone play a critical role in regulating skeletal growth, in promoting attaining peak bone mass and in

protecting against bone loss during adult life. Sex hormone deficiency in adulthood is associated with increased bone loss, because of increased bone remodelling and relative uncoupling between bone resorption and formation. Whilst bone cells express receptors for both oestrogens and androgens, the mechanisms by which sex hormones regulate bone turnover are incompletely understood. There is evidence to suggest that sex hormone deficiency causes increased production of cytokines such as tumour necrosis factor, interleukins-1 and -6, and M-CSF in the bone micro-environment, and that these stimulate bone resorption and cause uncoupling of bone formation.[29] Other mechanisms of sex hormone action that have also been proposed including an effect on the set point at which PTH is secreted, effects on calcitonin secretion, and effects on calcium absorption and calcitriol production. There is some evidence to suggest that the effects of testosterone on bone in males may be mediated in part by peripheral conversion to oestrogen by aromatase, which is expressed in adipose tissue and osteoblasts.[30]

Diet

Diet plays an important role in the attainment of peak bone mass and in maintaining skeletal health during adulthood.[31] The best studied nutrient is dietary calcium. High dietary calcium intakes during growth and adolescence have been associated with increased bone mass in various studies.[32] An adequate intake of calcium also appears to be important in preventing age-related bone loss, since calcium supplements in postmenopausal women have been shown to slow bone loss.[33] The protective effects of calcium on the skeleton in adults are probably mediated in part by a reduction in bone turnover due to suppression of parathyroid hormone (PTH) secretion, which normally increases with age. Other nutrients such as zinc, potassium, magnesium and fibre have also been associated with higher bone mass in epidemiological studies, although the mechanism responsible remains unclear. Energy intake is also related to bone mass, with effects that are partly mediated by changes in body weight. An extreme example of this is in anorexia nervosa, which can be associated with severe osteoporosis, although this is due in part to coexisting hypogonadism.[34]

Exercise

Exercise increases bone mass whereas immobility causes bone loss. The anabolic effects of exercise on bone mass seem to be most marked during growth and adolescence, although intense physical exercise has also been shown to have a positive effect on bone mass in adults.[35] Exercise has to involve high impact loading to be effective at increasing bone mass in adults. Moderate exercise does not increase bone mass significantly, but does improve muscle strength and balance, which is beneficial by reducing the likelihood of falls. Paradoxically, highly trained athletes such as marathon runners actually have reduced bone mass. This is due to the fact that the beneficial effects of skeletal loading are counterbalanced by low body weight and hypogonadism, both of which have detrimental effects on the skeleton.[36]

Smoking

Cigarette smokers are at increased risk of osteoporosis because of an earlier menopause, reduced body weight and altered metabolism of sex hormones (Table 4). Smokers also have an accelerated metabolism of exogenous oestrogens and impaired peripheral conversion of adrenal androgens to oestrogen. The conversion of adrenal androgens to oestrogen is particularly important postmenopausally, which may explain why the relative risk of hip fracture in female smokers increases progressively with age.[37]

Alcohol

Moderate alcohol intake does not seem to affect bone mass significantly, but chronic alcoholics are at increased risk of developing symptomatic osteoporosis. This is multifactorial in nature and probably occurs as the result of a direct inhibitory effect of alcohol on osteoblasts, coupled with indirect effects mediated by hypogonadism, relative immobility and poor diet.[38]

Table 4. Effects of smoking that increase risk of osteoporosis
Earlier menopause
Reduced body weight
Altered metabolism of sex hormones
Accelerated metabolism of exogenous oestrogens
Impaired peripheral conversion of adrenal androgens to oestrogen

Other risk factors

High caffeine intake has been linked to reduced bone mass and fractures in some studies, but not in others. On balance, it is unlikely to have a significant effect on the risk of osteoporosis. Pregnancy is associated with increased bone turnover and a reduction in bone mass which increases towards term and persists during lactation Thereafter, bone mass increases once again to return towards normal.[39]

Diseases and drugs associated with osteoporosis

In addition to the genetic and environmental factors mentioned above, osteoporosis can occur as a complication of various diseases and drug treatments. These are listed in Table 5 and are discussed in detail below.

Chronic inflammatory disease

Inflammatory diseases such as rheumatoid arthritis, ankylosing spondylitis, Crohn's disease and ulcerative colitis are all associated with an increased risk of osteoporosis.[40] This is multifactorial in nature and involves relative immobility; increased production of pro-inflammatory cytokines such as interleukin-1 and tumour necrosis factor, which stimulate bone resorption; and corticosteroid treatment, which suppresses bone formation. Malabsorption may also contribute to osteoporosis in patients with Crohn's disease.[41]

Table 5. Diseases and drugs associated with osteoporosis

Inflammatory disease	Miscellaneous
Rheumatoid arthritis	Haemoglobinopathy
Ankylosing spondylitis	Gaucher's disease
Inflammatory bowel disease	Myeloma
	Systemic mastocytosis
Gastrointestinal diseases	**Genetic diseases**
Coeliac disease	Osteogenesis imperfecta
Chronic pancreatitis	Osteoporosis–pseudoglioma syndrome
Chronic liver disease	Aromatase deficiency
Cystic fibrosis	Oestrogen receptor mutations
Endocrine diseases	**Drugs**
Hypogonadism	Corticosteroids
Thyrotoxicosis	GnRH agonists
Hyperparathyroidism	Thyroxine
Cushing's syndrome	Aromatase inhibitors
	Anticonvulsants
	Anticoagulants
	Sedatives

Gastrointestinal disease

Coeliac disease is associated with both osteoporosis and osteomalacia due to reduced intestinal absorption of calcium, vitamin D and other nutrients.[42] Osteoporosis may also occur as a complication of malabsorption in other diseases, such as chronic pancreatitis and cystic fibrosis.

Thyrotoxicosis

Thyrotoxicosis and over-replacement with thyroxine are both associated with reduced bone mass because of the stimulatory effects of thyroid hormone on bone turnover.[43] Epidemiological studies have shown that the risk of osteoporotic fractures is also increased in patients with a history of thyrotoxicosis.[44]

Primary hyperparathyroidism

Untreated primary hyperparathyroidism can be associated with increased loss and osteoporosis, especially in postmenopausal women.[45] This is thought to be due to the stimulatory effects of PTH on bone turnover combined with relative uncoupling of bone resorption from bone formation because of oestrogen deficiency.

Hypogonadism

Hypogonadism is the single most important cause of osteoporosis. Hypogonadism may be "physiological" as in postmenopausal osteoporosis, or pathological as in patients with early menopause, pituitary disease and gonadal failure due to infections, chemotherapy, or Turner's and Kleinfelter's syndromes. The mechanisms of osteoporosis include failure to attain peak bone mass (in Turner's and Kleinfelter's syndromes) and accelerated bone loss.

Corticosteroids

Corticosteroid treatment is an extremely important cause of osteoporosis in clinical practice (Table 6).[46] Corticosteroids cause osteoporosis by affecting several aspects of bone cell function and calcium homeostasis.[47] They inhibit intestinal calcium absorption, probably by antagonizing the effects of vitamin D on the gut. They also cause an increase in urinary calcium excretion by depressing renal tubular calcium absorption and reduce bone formation by inhibiting osteoblast activity. The direct effects of steroids on bone, gut and kidney cause a reduction in serum calcium, which in turn stimulates PTH secretion. The raised levels of PTH tend to restore serum calcium values towards normal, but this occurs partly at the expense of increasing bone resorption. This increase in resorption, when coupled with suppressed osteoblast activity, causes accelerated bone loss and, ultimately, osteoporosis. The risk of steroid-induced osteoporosis is related to the dose and duration of

Table 6. Effects of corticosteroid treatment that increase risk of osteoporosis
Inhibits intestinal calcium absorption
Increases urinary calcium loss
Reduces bone formation
Causes secondary hyperparathyroidism
Causes hypogonadism

therapy, although controversy exists as to whether or not there is a "safe" dose of steroids, since even low doses (<7.5 mg prednisolone per day) have been associated with increased rates of bone loss in some studies. Inhaled corticosteroids are less likely to cause osteoporosis than oral steroids, but may do so, especially when high doses are used on a long-term basis.

Other drugs

Long-acting benzodiazepines are associated with an increased risk of osteoporotic fracture, presumably because of their adverse effects on balance and cognitive function.[44] Anticonvulsant therapy is also associated with an increase in risk of osteoporotic fracture, although it is unclear if this is a direct effect on the skeleton or the result of coexisting risk factors in patients who require such treatment.[44] Gonadotrophin-releasing hormone agonists, used in the treatment of endometriosis and prostate cancer, cause osteoporosis by causing hypogonadism.[48] Prolonged heparin therapy is commonly considered to be a cause of osteoporosis, but there is actually little direct evidence to show that it actually does so.

Investigation and Diagnosis of Osteoporosis

Clinical assessment

Most patients with osteoporosis have no specific clinical signs, apart from kyphosis, which may be seen in patients with advanced vertebral osteoporosis. There are many causes for kyphosis other than osteoporosis, and the diagnosis of osteoporosis as the cause must be confirmed by demonstrating vertebral fractures on lateral spine radiographs. Clinical risk factors for osteoporosis can be identified on history taking and these provide a simple way to identify patients who need further investigation by bone densitometry (Table 7). Clinical evaluation may also uncover evidence of diseases that predispose to osteoporosis, such as thyrotoxicosis, hypogonadism and Cushing's syndrome. The presence of blue sclerae or a history of multiple fractures starting in childhood suggests a diagnosis of either osteogenesis imperfecta or one of the rare genetic syndromes associated with osteoporosis.

Bone densitometry

Bone densitometry is the investigation of first choice in the assessment of patients who are thought to be at risk of osteoporosis. Several technologies have been developed with which to measure bone density, but the two in most common use are dual energy X-ray absorptiometry (DEXA) and quantitative computed tomography (QCT) (Table 8). Both are based on the principle that calcium in bone mineral attenuates the passage of X-rays through bone tissue.

Measurements of BMD at the spine and hip (central DEXA) are considered the "gold standard" for the diagnosis of osteoporosis. Advantages of DEXA include a low radiation dose, high precision and rapid scanning time. The popularity of DEXA as a diagnostic tool stems from two factors. First, there is a strong correlation between BMD values as measured

Table 7. Indications for bone densitometry	
Sex hormone deficiency	Early menopause (<45 years)*
	Secondary amenorrhoea (>1 year)
	Hypogonadism
	Anorexia nervosa
Coexisting disease	Primary hyperparathyroidism
	Chronic inflammatory disease
	Malabsorption
	Organ transplantation
	Immobilization
Drug therapy	Corticosteroids (prednisolone >7.5 mg/day for > 3 months)
	GnRH agonists
Clinical evidence of osteoporosis	Radiological osteopaenia
	Previous fragility fracture
Clinical risk factors	Low body weight (BMI <20)
	Smoking
	Heavy alcohol intake
	Family history of hip fracture

*In the USA, BMD measurements are considered to be indicated in all postmenopausal women over the age of 65.

by DEXA and the occurrence of osteoporotic fractures (Figure 11). Second, information from randomized controlled trials of osteoporotic treatment have shown that the efficacy of bisphosphonates in preventing osteoporotic fracture is greatest in patients with low BMD as assessed by central DEXA.

Measurements made using QCT provide an alternative to DEXA. These provide a measure of true volumetric BMD, as well as distinguishing cortical BMD from trabecular BMD. QCT has a high radiation dose however and is less precise than DEXA, especially when used for trabecular measurements.

Table 8. Main methods of bone densitometry

Dual energy X-ray absorptiometry (DEXA)

Low radiation dose

High precision

Rapid scanning time

Strong correlation between measured BMD values and occurrence of osteoporotic fractures

Central DEXA can identify patients who will benefit most from bisphosphonate treatment

Quantitative computed tomography (QCT)

High radiation dose

Less precision than DEXA

Measures true volumetric BMD

Distinguishes cortical BMD from trabecular BMD

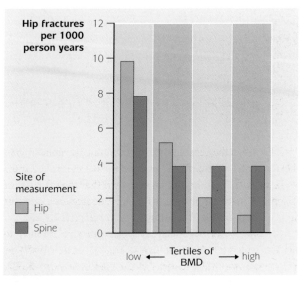

Figure 11. Prediction of hip fractures by bone densitometry. Adapted with permission from Elsevier Science from Cummings SR *et al*. Bone density at various sites for prediction of hip fractures. The Study of Osteoporotic Fractures Research Group. *Lancet* 1993; **341**: 72–75.[49]

A number of smaller DEXA and QCT devices, seemingly more suitable for a primary care physician's office, but with limited capability, are available at less cost than central DEXA and QCT methods. DEXA instruments are available for BMD measurement at the forearm, the heel and the finger, while a peripheral QCT (pQCT) instrument is available for measurement of BMD in the forearm. Peripheral densitometry has recently been shown in a large study in the United States to reliably predict the risk of sustaining an osteoporotic fracture.[50] However, there is limited information about the value of these technologies in targeting anti-osteoporotic treatment.

Whatever technology is used, densitometers give results as a function of the number of standard deviations by which the measured BMD value differs from the population mean, resulting in the so-called T-score and Z-score values (Figure 12). The T-score is a measure of how many standard deviations the patient's value deviates from young healthy individuals who have attained peak bone mass, whereas the Z-score value gives an estimate of how many standard deviations the measurement differs from age-matched controls. An example of the difference between T-score and Z-score values is

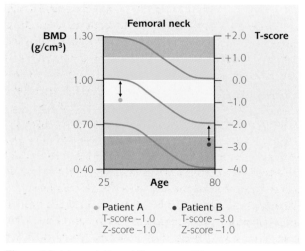

Figure 12. Interpretation of T-scores and Z-scores.

illustrated in Figure 12, which shows the results of hip DEXA analysis in two patients, one aged 33 years (A) and another aged 75 (B). Patient A has a Z-score of -1.0 and a T-score of -1.0. Both are within the normal range for the patient's age. Patient B has a Z-score of -1.0 and a T-score of -3.0. In this case, the BMD is 'normal' for the patient's age, but is in the osteoporotic range.

The predictive value of bone densitometry for fractures is similar to that for blood pressure and stroke, and three times better than that for cholesterol and acute myocardial infarction. Whilst BMD gives a good indication of risk in populations, the sensitivity and specificity at predicting fractures in the individual patient are not good enough to justify population-based BMD screening. Accordingly, bone densitometry is currently used as a diagnostic tool in selected patients with clinical risk factors of osteoporosis.

Quantitative ultrasound

Quantitative ultrasound (QUS) can also be used to evaluate the risk of osteoporotic fracture. Ultrasound examination is usually conducted at the heel, although devices have been developed which can analyse ultrasound properties of bone at other sites, such as the tibia and phalanges. Ultrasound results are usually expressed in terms of three parameters: broadband ultrasound attenuation (BUA), speed of sound (SOS) and stiffness, which is a composite measure, derived from an integration of BUA and SOS (Table 9). BUA values reflect the attenuation of sound waves as they pass through bone tissue and are proportionate to the density of the tissue. SOS values reflect the speed at which the sound waves travel through bone. These are related to BUA values but also provide a measure of tissue elasticity. Although ultrasound gives readings that are related to bone mass, it also assesses aspects of bone quality and structure that are not captured by BMD measurements. Of clinical relevance is the fact that ultrasound examination gives information that is complementary to, and additive with, bone mass measurements in the assessment of fracture risk (Figure 13). Most ultrasound machines give readouts expressed

Table 9. Expression of ultrasound results

Parameter	Comments
Broadband ultrasound attenuation (BUA)	The attenuation of sound waves as they pass through bone
	Proportionate to the density of the tissue
Speed of sound (SOS)	Speed at which sound waves travel through bone
	Thought to reflect tissue elasticity
Stiffness	Composite measure, derived from the integration of BUA and SOS

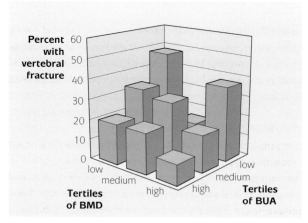

Figure 13. Combination of BMD and ultrasound to predict fractures. Adapted from Bauer DC *et al*. Quantitative ultrasound and vertebral fracture in postmenapausal women. Fracture Intervention Trial Research Group. *J Bone Miner Res* 1995; **10**: 353–358[51] with permission of the American Society for Bone and Mineral Research.

in terms of T-score and Z-score, allowing the clinician to relate the patient's value to age- and sex-matched controls. The difficulty with ultrasound devices is that they cannot be used

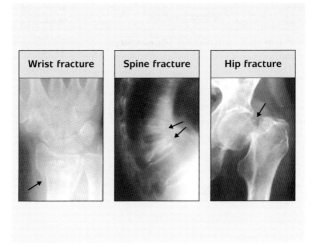

Figure 14. Common osteoporotic fractures.

to make a diagnosis of osteoporosis. However, as noted above, they can reliably be used to identify individuals who are at risk of osteoporotic fractures. Information is limited upon how QUS results should be used in deciding upon which patients to treat.

Radiographic examination

The principal application of radiographic examination is in the assessment of patients suspected to have fractures (Figure 14). Radiographs have poor sensitivity for the detection and monitoring of osteoporosis, since a large amount of bone mineral (over 30%) must be lost from the skeleton before it can be reliably detected on X-ray. Nonetheless, radiographic evidence of osteopaenia, when present, has been found to be a strong predictor of low BMD.[52] When a fracture is suspected on clinical grounds, radiographs should be taken of the affected bone in at least two planes at right angles to one another, and the films carefully examined for evidence of discontinuity in the bone cortex. In the vast majority of cases, plain radiographs are all that are required to confirm or refute a diagnosis of fracture. The diagnosis of vertebral fractures is also based on standard radiography and looking for subjective evidence of vertebral deformity. Increasingly, however, objective morphometric criteria are being used in the diagnosis and classification of vertebral fractures, especially in clinical trials. Using such criteria, vertebral fractures are defined to exist when there is more than a 20% loss of height between the anterior, middle or posterior aspects of the vertebral body on a lateral radiograph, or more than a 20% global reduction in height of one vertebra compared with the adjacent vertebrae. Recent evidence suggests that these "morphometric" vertebral fractures are positively correlated with back pain and morbidity, suggesting that they are clinically relevant.[53]

Other imaging techniques

Imaging with CT and MRI is seldom required in the investigation of osteoporosis. These techniques can be employed when plain radiographs are normal but clinical suspicion of a fracture remains high, or used to differentiate pathological fractures of the spine due to tumour deposits from fractures due to osteoporosis. Radionuclide bone scanning can also be helpful in the investigation of osteoporotic patients, particularly in differentiating bone pain due to fragility fractures from bone pain due to other causes, such as metastatic bone disease and Paget's disease. Bone scanning may also be useful in assessing whether a vertebral fracture is "new" (within the last 2 years) or the result of some long-forgotten trauma.

Bone turnover markers

Bone turnover can be assessed biochemically by measuring serum and/or urine levels of factors that are secreted by osteoblasts during bone formation or released from bone matrix during bone resorption (Table 10). The most commonly used markers of bone resorption are those which measure collagen cross-links that are released from bone when it is resorbed by osteoclast activity. It is possible to measure levels of the free cross-links that join collagen molecules (pyridinoline or deoxypyridinoline), or cross-links which remain attached to the N- and C-terminal fragments of the collagen chain

Table 10. Biochemical markers of bone turnover in routine use

	Marker type	Derived from
Bone resorption	Urine deoxypyridinoline	Bone collagen degradation
	Urine or serum collagen telopeptides (CTX, NTX)	Bone collagen degradation
Bone formation	Serum total alkaline phosphatase	Osteoblasts/liver/kidney
	Serum bone-specific alkaline phosphatase	Osteoblasts
	Serum osteocalcin	Osteoblasts
	Serum collagen pro-peptides (PINP, PICP)	Released during collagen synthesis

(telopeptide cross-links, NTX and CTX). Two broad categories of bone formation marker are in current use: proteins which are released from osteoblasts such as osteocalcin and alkaline phosphatase, and fragments of collagen pro-peptides which are cleaved from collagen during matrix deposition.

Biochemical markers reflect bone turnover, and elevated levels of some markers have been found to predict fracture risk (Figure 15). They cannot be used in the diagnosis of osteoporosis, since elevated levels are a non-specific finding in patients with recent fracture and other metabolic bone diseases associated with increased bone turnover. The clinical utility of biochemical markers as a way of assessing treatment response and compliance is currently being explored, although this largely remains a research-based technique at present.

Genetic markers

The importance of heredity in the pathogenesis of osteoporosis opens up the possibility that genetic markers could be used to identify patients at risk of fractures. Genetic markers of fracture risk are starting to be developed for clinical use. One marker which is commercially available (COLIA1 GenotypR™)

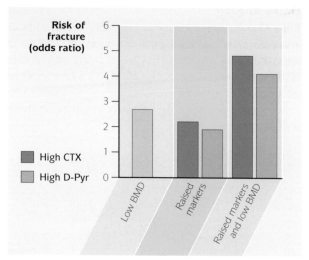

Figure 15. Combination of biochemical markers and BMD to predict fractures. Reproduced with permission from Garrero P, Harsherr E, Chapuy ML et al. J Bone Min Res 1996; **11**: 1531–1538. [54]

detects an Sp1 binding site polymorphism in the COLIA1 gene which has been found to be associated with osteoporotic fractures in several population-based studies and case control studies. Current data indicate that the relative risk of fracture is increased by about 50% for each copy of the unfavourable allele detected by this test.[25]

Routine biochemistry and haematology

A routine biochemical and haematological screen, including assessment of thyroid function, liver function tests, calcium biochemistry, serum proteins, full blood count and erythrocyte sedimentation rate (ESR), should be performed to screen for secondary causes of osteoporosis. Serum oestradiol and gonadotrophins should be checked in young women with osteoporosis who are amenorrhoeic or oligomenorrhoeic, but these tests are not necessary in women who have straightforward postmenopausal osteoporosis.

Bone biopsy

Bone biopsies are not required to make a diagnosis of osteoporosis, but can be helpful in determining the underlying cause. Bone biopsies are of most help in young patients with severe osteoporosis where the cause is unclear or when osteomalacia is suspected.

A suggested diagnostic algorithm for osteoporosis is shown in Figure 16.

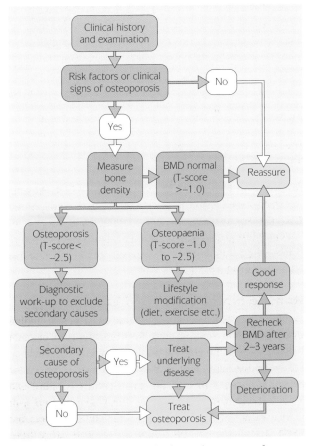

Figure 16. Algorithm for investigation and treatment of osteoporosis.

Prevention of Osteoporosis

Here, we will discuss lifestyle modifications and drug treatments which have been used to prevent postmenopausal bone loss and those which have been used for the primary prevention of osteoporotic fractures.

There has been much debate as to the cost effectiveness of strategies aimed at the primary prevention of bone loss. Public health measures aimed at improving diet, increasing exercise and modifying risk factors for osteoporosis are being used in many countries, but the impact which these have on the burden of fractures is difficult to ascertain. Drug treatments are available that are highly effective for the prevention of postmenopausal bone loss, but it is not clear how they should best be used in routine clinical practice. Bone loss is an invariable occurrence in postmenopausal women and, in over 50% of cases, will eventually lead to the development of osteoporosis. Unfortunately, it is not possible to identify women who will develop osteoporosis at the time of menopause and, even if this were possible, it would not be cost effective to administer anti-osteoporotic drugs to large sections of the population for up to 30 years simply to prevent BMD values falling below the T-score of −2.5. At present, therefore, drug treatment is seldom given for the primary prevention of bone loss in patients whose initial BMD values are normal.

The situation is different for the primary prevention of fragility fractures. Here, treatments can be effectively targeted to individuals at high risk on the basis that they already have low BMD. Currently, primary prevention is given to two main patient groups: postmenopausal women with BMD T-scores of −2.5 or below, and elderly men and women who are at risk of hip fracture because of low BMD or other risk factors. The treatment options for primary prevention of bone loss and osteoporotic fractures are discussed individually in more detail below and summarized in Table 11.

Diet

Patients who are identified to be at risk of osteoporosis because of low bone density or clinical risk factors should be advised to take a balanced diet with an adequate protein, energy, calcium and vitamin D intake. The recommended calcium intake for premenopausal women and men is 1000 mg daily and that for postmenopausal women 1500 mg daily. Since dairy products are the richest source of dietary calcium, men would require about 1 pint of milk daily and women 1.5 pints of milk daily to reach this target. Individuals with osteoporosis or osteopaenia who are taking less than this amount and are unable or unwilling to increase consumption of dairy products should be advised to take calcium supplements. While calcium is important for maintaining skeletal health, as a single agent it has been shown to be ineffective in preventing early

Table 11. Treatment options for the prevention of bone loss and primary prevention of osteoporotic fractures

Treatment	Effect on BMD	Effect on vertebral fracture	Effect on non-vertebral fracture
Exercise[58]	Yes	nt	nt
Increase dietary calcium[57]	Yes	nt	nt
Calcium[55,61]	Yes	Yes	Yes
Calcium and vitamin D[66-68]	Yes	Yes	Yes
HRT[69-71,74]	Yes	Yes	Yes
Raloxifene[77,78]	Yes	Yes	No
Tibolone[80]	Yes	nt	nt
Cyclical etidronate[82]	Yes	nt	nt
Alendronate[83-86]	Yes	Yes	Yes
Risedronate[89,90]	Yes	nt	Yes

nt – not tested for this indication

postmenopausal bone loss except in women with very low calcium intakes of 400 mg/day or less.[55] Vitamin D deficiency is another important factor in the pathogenesis of osteoporotic hip fractures, and those at risk of deficiency include elderly housebound subjects and those in institutional care. Such individuals should be encouraged to take a diet with adequate amounts of vitamin D-containing foods such as dairy products and meat, and if this is not possible, supplementation should be given in the form of multivitamin tablets or cod liver oil. Epidemiological studies have shown a positive association between intake of dairy products during skeletal growth and peak bone mass in adulthood. Clinical trials have convincingly shown that calcium or milk supplementation increases bone mass in children and adolescents,[56] and slows bone loss in postmenopausal women.[57] These observations emphasize the importance of taking a diet rich in calcium and vitamin D during bone growth, as well as in adulthood.

Exercise

Physical exercise has been shown to have a preventative effect on bone loss. A meta-analysis of randomized trials in this area[58] showed that exercise involving impact loading increased spine BMD by a mean (95% CI) of 1.6% (1.0–2.2%) compared with controls, whereas non-impact exercise increased BMD by 1% (0.4–1.6%). Corresponding values for femoral neck BMD were 0.9% (0.5–1.3%) and 1.4% (0.2–2.6%). The effects of exercise on osteoporotic fracture have not been studied in the context of a randomized trial, but several investigators have found that muscle strength and physical activity are inversely related to the risk of vertebral and non-vertebral osteoporotic fractures (Figure 17).[59] Although these beneficial effects of exercise on fracture incidence could be partly due to changes in BMD, they seem more likely to be attributable to improved muscle strength and a reduced risk of falling. Physical exercise should therefore be encouraged in patients who are at risk of osteoporotic fractures. Physical exercise during skeletal growth is also beneficial for the skeleton; several investigators have found that regular weight-bearing exercise during childhood

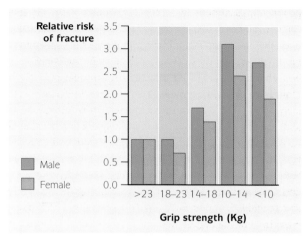

Figure 17. Effect of muscle strength on the risk of hip fracture. Reproduced with permission from Lau E *et al.* Physical activity and calcium intake in fracture of the proximal femur in Hong Kong. *Br Med J* 1988; **297**: 1441–1443.[59]

and adolescence is positively associated with peak bone mass.[60] This emphasizes the importance of encouraging physical exercise to promote bone health in the young as well as old.

Smoking, alcohol and other factors

Patients at risk of osteoporosis should be strongly advised to stop smoking from the point of view of their bones and their general health, in view of its association with reduced BMD, early menopause and osteoporotic fracture. Those with a heavy alcohol intake (>20 units/week in women and 30 units/week in men) should be advised to cut down, but moderate alcohol intake can be continued without adversely affecting osteoporosis. Benzodiazepines should be stopped wherever possible, since elderly patients who are receiving such treatment have an increased risk of fracture, presumably because they are at increased risk of falling. Replacement therapy with thyroxine should be adjusted to maintain TSH levels within the normal range, since thyroxine over-replacement has been associated with low BMD, presumably because it stimulates bone turnover. Reduced visual acuity is also associated with and increased risk of fracture, and patients with this problem should be referred to the appropriate specialists for advice and treatment.

Calcium and vitamin D

Calcium supplements of between 1000 and 2000 mg daily slow bone loss in postmenopausal women by suppressing PTH secretion and reducing bone turnover. As might be expected, the response to calcium supplements have been found to be greatest in people with a low calcium intake, but benefits have also been observed in subjects with normal dietary calcium.[33,55,61] Some investigators have also found that the response of BMD is related to vitamin D receptor genotype.[62] Calcium supplements have also been shown in some primary prevention studies to reduce the risk of vertebral and non-vertebral fractures.[61] Vitamin D supplementation without additional calcium has been found to reduce bone loss in elderly women.[63,64] These effects are also mediated by suppressing PTH secretion and have been found to be related to vitamin D receptor (VDR) genotype.[65] Combinations of calcium and vitamin D supplements have been found to reduce the risk of fractures in older people in randomized controlled trials. Dawson-Hughes et al. treated 176 men and 213 women aged 65 and over with femoral neck BMD values below –2.0 with 700 IU vitamin D plus 500 mg calcium daily, or placebo. The rate of non-vertebral fractures was decreased by about 50% in the calcium and vitamin D group after 3 years treatment.[66] In another study, Chapuy et al. treated 3270 elderly women of average age 84 years with 800 IU vitamin D plus 1.2 g calcium, or placebo.[67,68] The treatment increased BMD and reduced the rate of non-vertebral fractures by about 30% (Figure 18). The administration of vitamin D supplements to elderly individuals in the absence of calcium supplements has not been found to be effective in preventing fractures.[63] In summary, calcium and vitamin D supplementation, when combined, seem to be more effective than either agent alone in the prevention of bone loss and in the primary prevention of osteoporotic non-vertebral fractures in the elderly.

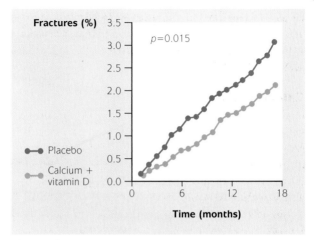

Figure 18. Effects of calcium and vitamin D on non-vertebral fractures in elderly women. Adapted with permission from Chapuy MC *et al.* Vitamin D3 and calcium to prevent hip fractures in the elderly woman. *New Engl J Med* 1992; **327**: 1637–1642.[68] Copyright © 2002 Massachusetts Medical Society.

Hormone replacement therapy

Hormone replacement therapy (HRT) is a highly effective treatment for the prevention of postmenopausal bone loss, and has also been shown to prevent height loss and osteoporotic fractures (Figure 19).[69–71] The inhibitory effects of HRT on bone loss are probably mediated for the most part by a direct action on bone cells, although secondary changes in calcium-regulating hormones may also contribute, since HRT has been found to increase intestinal calcium absorption, serum 1,25-hydroxyvitamin D_3 levels and to suppress PTH levels.[72] HRT can be given in the form of oestrogen alone to patients who have had a hysterectomy, but progestagens should be added in women with an intact uterus to reduce the risk of endometrial carcinoma. Progestagens may either be given sequentially with oestrogen to mimic the normal menstrual cycle or continuously on a combined basis. Continuous combined HRT does not cause resumption of regular menstrual bleeding, but breakthrough bleeding is quite common,

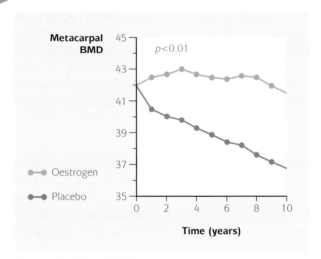

Figure 19. Effect of HRT on bone mass after oophorectomy.
Adapted with permission from Elsevier Science from Lindsay R *et al*. Prevention of spinal osteoporosis in oophorectomised women. *Lancet* 1980; **ii**: 1151–1154.[71]

especially during the early stages of therapy. Many formulations of HRT are available, but there is no direct evidence to suggest that one has any clear advantage over another as regards the skeletal response, so long as the dose of oestrogen is adequate. Absolute contraindications to HRT include breast cancer, endometrial cancer and venous thromboembolism, whereas immobilization, recent surgery and a personal or family history of venous thromboembolism are relative contraindications. In addition to its beneficial effects on bone, HRT improves vasomotor symptoms and atrophic vaginitis, which are themselves important indications for therapy in perimenopausal women.

What about the adverse effects of HRT? Meta-analysis of epidemiological data indicate that the risk of breast cancer may be increased by up to 30% in long-term HRT users (>15 years).[73] This is an important disincentive to starting HRT therapy for many women. A recent large scale study has confirmed that HRT increases the risk of breast cancer when administered to healthy postmenopausal women and increases the risk of coronary heart disease, DVT and stroke. This is partly offset by a reduced risk of hip fracture and breast cancer. However, overall the effect of HRT on mortality in this study was neutral.[74] A relatively short-term study looking at the effect of HRT in the secondary prevention of coronary heart disease in women (HERS study) showed no overall effect of HRT in terms of cardiovascular mortality.[75] An important limitation of HRT in the prevention of osteoporosis is adherence to treatment. Although the uptake rate of HRT is initially high in the early postmenopausal years, few patients remain on treatment in the long term. This is relevant since the protective effect of HRT on fractures is strongest in women who are current users, and wears off rapidly after treatment is stopped.[76]

Raloxifene

Raloxifene belongs to a class of agents termed selective oestrogen receptor modulators (SERMs), which are drugs that act as oestrogen agonists in some tissues and oestrogen antagonists in others. Raloxifene (Evista™) has been found in large randomized controlled trials to inhibit bone turnover, increase bone mass and to prevent the risk of vertebral fractures in postmenopausal women with low bone density. Randomized controlled dose-ranging studies have shown that raloxifene in doses of 30, 60 and 150 mg daily increases bone mass at the spine, hip and total body by about 2–3% over a 2-year treatment period when compared to persons receiving only calcium and vitamin D.[77] Raloxifene also lowers serum levels of cholesterol, due mainly to an effect on low-density lipoprotein. Raloxifene has been shown to be an effective agent for the primary prevention of vertebral fractures in a large randomized controlled trial. Raloxifene in doses of 60 and 120 mg was given to 7705 postmenopausal women with low BMD, along with calcium and vitamin D supplements. Both doses increased BMD and reduced the incidence of vertebral, but not non-vertebral, fractures over a 3-year treatment period, when compared with calcium- and vitamin D-supplemented placebo.[78] In this study, raloxifene treatment was associated with an increased risk of venous thromboembolic disease [relative risk 3.1 (1.5–6.2)], but a reduced risk of breast cancer [relative risk 0.24 (0.13–0.44)].[79] Raloxifene is generally well tolerated; the only side-effect noted more commonly in raloxifene-treated patients compared with placebo-treated patients in randomized controlled trials was hot flushes, which occurred 7% more frequently in raloxifene-treated patients than in the placebo-treated patients.

Tamoxifen (Nolvadex™), which is widely used in the prevention and treatment of breast cancer and can be regarded as a SERM, also prevents bone loss in oestrogen-deficient women.

Tibolone

Tibolone (Livial™) is a steroid hormone which acts as a partial agonist at the oestrogen, progesterone and androgen receptors. Tibolone in doses of 1.25–2.5 mg daily has been found to increase spine bone mass by about 5% and wrist bone mass by 1–2% in postmenopausal women.[80] Tibolone is also effective at alleviating vasomotor symptoms and acts to enhance libido, without causing endometrial stimulation.[81] The effects of tibolone on lipid profile have been mixed. Tibolone reduces levels of HDL cholesterol, but also decreases total cholesterol and triglycerides. The long-term effects on clinically relevant cardiovascular endpoints such as myocardial infarction and stroke are unknown. Livial has not yet been shown to prevent the occurrence of osteoporotic fractures, but studies are ongoing at the moment to address this issue.

Bisphosphonates

Bisphosphonates are potent inhibitors of osteoclastic bone resorption. They share in common a core structure of phosphorus–carbon–phosphorus atoms to which are attached various side chains at the R_1 and R_2 positions (Figure 20). The phosphorus–carbon–phosphorus moiety targets bisphosphonate to the skeleton, where it accumulates at sites of increased bone turnover. When bone containing bisphosphonate is ingested by resorbing osteoclasts, the drug is released within the cell, thereby inhibiting osteoclast function. Three bisphosphonates

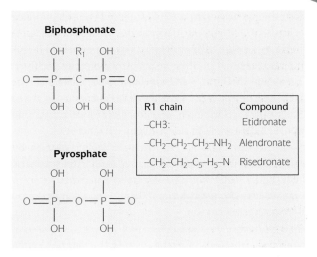

Figure 20. Structure of bisphosphonates.

are currently licensed in Europe for the prevention and treatment of osteoporosis – cyclical etidronate (Didronel PMO), alendronate (Fosamax) and risedronate (Actonel) – and two of these (alendronate and risedronate) are also licensed in North America.

Cyclical etidronate given in combination with calcium supplements has been found to increase bone mass when compared with calcium-supplemented placebo in early postmenopausal women.[82] The regimen involves taking oral etidronate in a dose of 400 mg daily for 14 days, followed by calcium supplementation of 500 mg daily for 76 days. Didronel PMO is well tolerated but the etidronate component needs to be given on an empty stomach, because intestinal absorption of the drug is poor and is inhibited further when taken with food. No data are available on the effects of Didronel PMO on primary prevention of vertebral and non-vertebral fractures.

Alendronate is an effective agent for the prevention of bone loss and the primary prevention of osteoporotic fractures in postmenopausal women. The effects of alendronate on bone loss were studied in a placebo-controlled trial of 1174 postmenopausal women aged 60 or under. When administered in doses of 2.5 and 5 mg daily, alendronate increased spine BMD by about 2–3%, whereas placebo-treated patients experienced a fall in BMD of 2%. At the femoral neck site, the gain in BMD was 1–2% with alendronate compared with a 1% loss in placebo.[83] Three other randomized controlled studies of 5–10 mg daily alendronate in postmenopausal women with low BMD showed consistent increases in bone mass at the spine and hip, and a reduced risk of vertebral and non-vertebral fractures (Figure 21).[84–86] In all of these studies, both alendronate- and placebo-treated patients received supplementation with calcium (500 mg) and vitamin D (250 IU) when dietary calcium was estimated as less than 1000 mg. An important finding to emerge from these studies was that the beneficial effects of alendronate on fracture prevention were limited to patients with osteoporosis, i.e. patients with BMD T-scores below –2.5.[85]

Recent studies have shown that alendronate (70 mg, once weekly) gives an equivalent increase in BMD to daily doses of 10 mg and has the advantage of being greatly preferred by patients.[87] No data are available on the effects of once weekly alendronate on fracture.

Alendronate must be given on an empty stomach with a large glass of water because absorption is inhibited by food. Alendronate has been found to be well tolerated in randomized controlled trials, with a safety profile similar to that of placebo. Gastrointestinal side-effects including oesophagitis have been reported in some patients taking alendronate.[88] These side-effects are most likely to occur in patients with pre-existing gastro-oesophageal reflux disease and when the medication has been taken incorrectly. Side-effects do not seem to be a common problem if the drug is used with caution in these patient groups and the dosing recommendations are adhered to. Problems with gastrointestinal intolerance seem to be slightly less common with weekly alendronate.[87]

Risedronate prevents bone loss in postmenopausal women[89] and has also been found to be effective in the primary prevention of hip fractures in older women.[90] A randomized placebo-

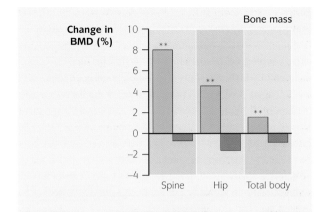

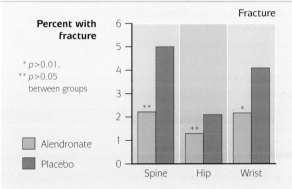

Figure 21. Effect of alendronate on bone mass and primary prevention of osteoporotic fracture in postmenopausal osteoporosis. Data from Liberman *et al*. Effect of oral alendronate on bone mineral density and the incidence of fractures in postmenapausal osteoporosis. The Alendronate Phase III Osteoporosis Treatment Study Group. *New Engl J Med* 1995; **333**: 1437–1443.[84]

controlled trial of daily 2.5 or 5 mg risedronate in postmenopausal women with low BMD (T-score less than –2.0) showed that both doses increased bone density when compared with placebo.[89] The effect was greatest with the 5 mg dose, which increased spine bone density by about 4% and femoral neck bone density by about 2%. Calcium supplements were given to all patients.

Another study looked at the effects of risedronate in the primary prevention of hip fracture in elderly subjects.[90] In this study, 2.5 or 5 mg risedronate was administered daily for 3 years to 9331 elderly women at risk of hip fracture. Two groups of women were enrolled into the study with different entry criteria; 5445 women aged 70–79 years were enrolled on the basis that they had low BMD alone (T-score < –4.0) or had low BMD (T-score < –3.0) and at least one clinical risk factor for hip fracture. The remaining 3886 subjects were enrolled on the basis that they were aged at least 80 years and had either a clinical risk factor or had low BMD alone. Calcium and vitamin D supplements were given to all patients. The study showed a 39% reduction in new hip fractures in the risedronate-treated patients when compared with the placebo group (Figure 22), although the beneficial effects were restricted to the younger patients, who were primarily enrolled on the basis that they had low BMD.

Like other bisphosphonates, risedronate must be given on an empty stomach with a large glass of water, because absorption is poor and is inhibited by food. Risedronate appears to be well tolerated, with a side-effect profile which is no different from placebo.

Agents in development

Zoledronate is a highly potent bisphosphonate that is used intravenously for the treatment of cancer-associated bone disease. Recent studies have shown that single injections of 4 mg increase BMD and suppress bone resorption for periods of up to 1 year (Figure 23).[91] Whilst this drug holds great promise, the effects on fracture are unknown. Ibandronate is another potent bisphosphonate which has also been given by injection in the prevention of osteoporosis.[92] A large randomized controlled trial showed that 3-monthly ibandronate (2 mg) increased BMD in patients with postmenopausal osteoporosis, but did not reduce the incidence of fractures. Evaluation of biochemical markers from this study showed that the treatment did not give sustained suppression of bone turnover, and further studies are in progress with different dose schedules to determine if anti-fracture efficacy can be demonstrated.

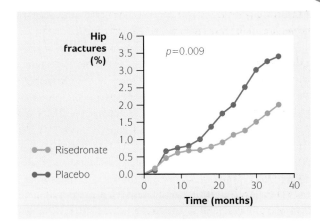

Figure 22. HIP trial with risedronate. Adapted with permission from McClung MR *et al*. Effect of risedronate on the risk of hip fracture in elderly women. *New Engl J Med* 2001; **344**: 333–340.[90] Copyright © 2002 Massachusetts Medical Society.

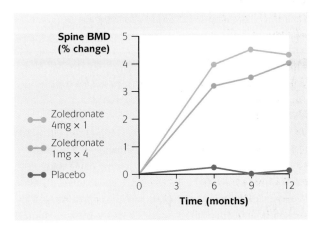

Figure 23. Once yearly injection of zoledronate increases BMD. Adapted with permission from Reid IR *et al*. Intravenous zoledronic acid in postmenopausal women with low bone mineral density. *New Engl J Med* 2002; **346**: 653–661.[91]Copyright © 2002 Massachusetts Medical Society.

Treatment of Established Osteoporosis

There is little doubt about the cost effectiveness of treating established osteoporosis, since patients with low BMD and fragility fractures are at high risk of future fractures.[93] This is especially true in osteoporotic patients who develop a vertebral fracture, where the risk of further fracture within 1 year is about 20%.[94] Many treatment options are available for the secondary prevention of osteoporotic fractures and some of these are also used in the prevention of osteoporosis. In this section, we focus on treatments which have been used for the secondary prevention of osteoporotic fractures. The evidence supporting the use of these agents is summarized in Table 12 and the individual therapies are discussed in more detail below.

Calcium and vitamin D

Calcium and vitamin D supplements should be given as baseline therapy in patients with established osteoporosis where dietary intake is suboptimal. Calcium and vitamin D supplements alone have limited anti-fracture efficacy in this situation and are usually used in combination with other agents.

Vitamin D metabolites

The active metabolites of vitamin D, 1α-hydroxyvitamin D (Alfacalcidol™) and 1,25-dihydroxyvitamin D (Rocaltrol™), have both been studied in the treatment of patients with established osteoporosis. The presumed mechanism of action is by increasing calcium absorption with suppression of PTH secretion, although there is some evidence from preclinical studies that low concentrations of 1,25-dihydroxyvitamin D can also inhibit osteoclast activity. In Japanese subjects, 1α-hydroxyvitamin D plus calcium supplements have been found to significantly reduce the rate of new fractures when compared with calcium supplements alone, although the effects of this

Table 12. Treatment options in patients with established osteoporosis

Treatment	Effect on BMD	Effect on vertebral fracture	Effect on non-vertebral fracture
Vitamin D metabolites[95-97]	Yes	Yes	No
Calcitonin[98]	Yes	Yes	No
Fluoride[99]	Yes	No	No
Raloxifene[78]	Yes	Yes	No
Cyclical etidronate[100, 101]	Yes	Yes	No
Alendronate[83-86, 109]	Yes	Yes	Yes
Risedronate[89, 90, 103, 104]	Yes	Yes	Yes
Parathyroid hormone[105]	Yes	Yes	Yes

metabolite on fracture have not been studied in other ethnic groups.[97] Studies of 1,25-dihydroxyvitamin D in Caucasians with established osteoporosis have yielded mixed results. In a double-blind RCT of 2 years duration, no beneficial effects on the secondary prevention of fractures was observed in 86 patients with established osteoporosis and vertebral fractures treated with 1,25-dihydroxyvitamin D (0.25–0.5 mcg) plus calcium supplements (1000 mg daily) versus calcium supplements alone.[95] In another study, 1,25-dihydroxyvitamin D (0.25 mcg daily) combined with calcium supplements (1 g daily) was found to significantly reduce the rate of new vertebral and non-vertebral fractures over a 3-year period in Caucasian patients when compared with calcium supplements alone.[96] The results of this study should be treated with caution, however, since 1,25-dihydroxyvitamin D treatment did not reduce the rate of fracture, and the significant difference between the groups was mainly attributable to the fact that patients receiving calcium supplements alone had a significant increase in the rate of fractures when compared with baseline.

Calcitonin

Calcitonin acts directly on mature osteoclasts to inhibit bone resorption, and has been shown to inhibit bone turnover and increase bone mass in postmenopausal women. Various formulations of calcitonin are available, but most recent research in the osteoporosis field has focused on intranasal calcitonin. The pivotal study of intranasal calcitonin in osteoporosis is the PROOF study,[98] which included 1255 women with established osteoporosis and vertebral fractures who were randomized to receive placebo or intranasal calcitonin in doses of 100, 200 and 400 IU daily over a 5-year treatment period. All patients received daily calcium (1 g daily) and vitamin D supplements (250 IU daily). The incidence of new vertebral fractures was reduced by calcitonin when data from all active treatment groups were combined, but subgroup analysis showed that the protective effect was restricted to the 200 IU dose. Although these data indicate that intranasal calcitonin may be effective in the prevention of vertebral fracture, the validity of the results from this study have been questioned in view of the fact that the drop-out rate was high (almost 60%) and the fact that there was no dose response. A meta-analysis of 14 clinical trials that compared intranasal or injectable calcitonin with placebo or no treatment in the prevention of osteoporotic fractures has also been published.[106] This showed that the relative risk of any fracture for individuals taking calcitonin was 0.43 (95% CI 0.38–0.50) when compared with subjects not taking calcitonin. The effect was apparent for both vertebral fracture (relative risk 0.45; 95% CI 0.39–0.53) and non-vertebral fractures (relative risk 0.34; 95% CI 0.17–0.68). Although this raises the possibility that calcitonin may prevent non-vertebral fractures, it is of concern that intranasal calcitonin did not protect against non-vertebral fracture significantly in the PROOF study.

The intranasal preparation of calcitonin is well tolerated and the only side-effect noted more frequently in patients receiving active treatment was rhinitis. There is some evidence to suggest that intranasal and injectable calcitonin has an analgaesic effect in patients with acute vertebral fracture,[107] but this has not been rigorously studied in large-scale randomized controlled trials.

Fluoride

Fluoride stimulates bone formation. The mechanism of action is incompletely understood, but the available evidence suggests that it inhibits protein phosphatases in osteoblasts, causing activation of osteoblast growth and increased matrix synthesis.[108] Treatment of osteoporotic patients with fluoride stimulates biochemical markers of bone formation and causes an increase in bone mass, whereas markers of bone resorption are unaffected. Several doses and formulations of fluoride have been used in the treatment of osteoporosis.[99] Sodium fluoride has been used in doses of about 10–40 mg daily and monofluorophosphate in doses of about 20–25 mg daily. In all studies, fluoride has been used in combination with calcium supplements or calcium and vitamin D supplements. Both formulations of fluoride have been shown to increase BMD in the lumbar spine in a dose-dependent manner, although no consistent stimulatory effect on BMD has been observed at sites rich in cortical bone, such as the hip and wrist. The effects of fluoride on fracture prevention have been mixed, and a recent meta-analysis of 12 RCTs performed between 1980 and 1998 showed no significant reduction in vertebral fractures or non vertebral fractures.[99] The main side-effects of fluoride to emerge from the meta-analysis of these studies was lower limb pain. In summary, the risk-benefit ratio of sodium fluoride in the treatment of established osteoporosis does not seem favourable, given the availability of other safer and more effective treatments.

Raloxifene

Raloxifene has also been shown to reduce the risk of vertebral fracture in postmenopausal women with established osteoporosis. The pivotal study of raloxifene in established

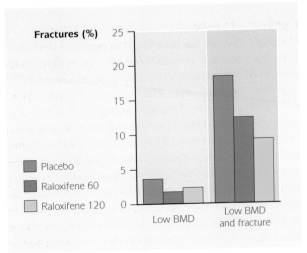

Figure 24. Effect of raloxifene on fractures. Adapted with permission from Ettinger B *et al*. Reduction of vertebral fracture risk in postmenopausal women with osteoporosis treated with raloxifene. *J Am Med Assoc* 1999; **282**: 637–645.[78]

osteoporosis is the MORE trial, which included 7705 postmenopausal women of average age 64 years.[78] Approximately 50% of participants in this study had established osteoporosis with one or more vertebral fractures at baseline. Raloxifene in doses of 60 and 120 mg daily increased bone density at the spine and hip by about 2–3%, and reduced the risk of vertebral fracture by 30% in patients given a 60 mg dose and 50% in patients given 120 mg. The anti-fracture effect of raloxifene was seen both in women who did and did not have prevalent fractures at baseline (Figure 24). Surprisingly, raloxifene had no significant effect on the prevention of non-vertebral fractures, although overall there was a significant reduction in ankle fractures and a trend towards reduction with some other fractures.

Cyclical etidronate

Cyclical etidronate has been found to increase spinal bone mass and prevent vertebral fractures in patients with established osteoporosis.[100, 101] In the study of Storm et al.,[100] etidronate increased spine BMD by about 5% and reduced the rate of new vertebral fractures during years 2–3 from 54 per 100 patient years to six per 100 patient years in a group of 66 women with established osteoporosis. Although this difference was significant, there was no significant difference between the groups over the 3-year study period. Another study conducted over 2 years by Watts et al.[101] compared the effects of cyclical etidronate and calcium, with and without phosphate therapy, with calcium-supplemented placebo in 429 patients with established osteoporosis. Phosphate had no effect on BMD or fracture in either the etidronate or placebo groups, so data from the phosphate- and non-phosphate-treated etidronate and placebo groups were combined in statistical analysis. The rate of new vertebral fractures was reduced by about 50% in the groups of patients who received etidronate when compared with those who received placebo, and subgroup analysis showed a 60% reduction in patients with the lowest BMD at baseline. An extension of this study for a third year showed an increase in fracture rate in the etidronate group, such that no significant benefit was observed when data for all three years were combined. Evidence from post-marketing surveillance studies in the UK indicate that etidronate might prevent the development of non-vertebral fractures,[102] but this has not been proven in the context of a randomized controlled study. Cyclical etidronate is well tolerated, but the available data indicate that it is less effective than other more potent bisphosphonates in the management of established osteoporosis.

Alendronate

Alendronate has been shown to increase bone density, inhibit bone turnover and reduce the incidence of vertebral and non-vertebral fractures in large-scale randomized trials. In the pivotal fracture intervention trial, 2027 women with low BMD and vertebral fractures were randomized to receive alendronate (10 mg daily) or placebo.[109] Calcium supplements were given to patients who had low dietary calcium in both groups. The rate of new vertebral fracture was reduced by 50% in alendronate-treated patients, and similar reductions were observed in wrist fracture and hip fractures. The recommended dose of alendronate for the treatment of established osteoporosis is 10 mg daily, or 70 mg once weekly. Calcium and vitamin D supplements should also be given to patients where dietary intake is suboptimal.

Risedronate

Risedronate has been shown to reduce bone turnover, increase bone density, and reduce the incidence of vertebral and non-vertebral fractures in large-scale randomized trials. Two pivotal studies of risedronate have been conducted in patients with established osteoporosis who had pre-existing vertebral fractures. In one study, 1226 women with established osteoporosis and two or more vertebral fractures were randomized to receive placebo or risedronate in doses of 2.5 or 5 mg daily.[103] All patients received calcium supplements (1 g), and vitamin D supplements (500 IU daily) were also given to patients where baseline 25-hydroxyvitamin D levels were low. The 5 mg dose significantly reduced the rate of new vertebral fractures by about 50% after 3 years. The 2.5 mg dose was similarly effective but treatment was stopped after 2 years due to a protocol amendment. In another study of similar design,[104] 2548 postmenopausal women with established osteoporosis and at least one vertebral fracture were randomized to receive placebo or risedronate in doses of 2.5 or 5 mg daily. The 2.5 mg dose was stopped after 1 year, but the 5 mg dose group showed a 41% reduction in vertebral fracture at 3 years and a 39% reduction in non-vertebral fractures.

The recommended dose of risedronate for the treatment of osteoporosis is 5 mg daily. Calcium and vitamin D supplements should also be given to patients where dietary intake is suboptimal. Risedronate is well tolerated and, in the large-

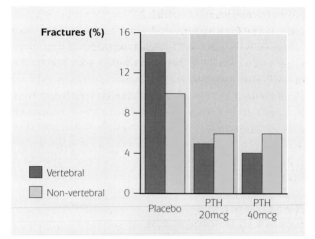

Figure 25. Effects of PTH on vertebral and non-vertebral fracture. Data from Neer RM *et al.* Effect of parathyroid hormone (1–34) on fractures and bone mineral density in postmenopausal women with osteoporosis. *New Engl J Med* 2001; **344**: 1434–1441.[105]

scale clinical trials that have been performed so far, the adverse effect profile has not been found to be different from placebo.

Parathyroid hormone

Parathyroid hormone (PTH) has been found to markedly increase bone mass and to dramatically reduce the risk of vertebral and non-vertebral fractures in postmenopausal women with established osteoporosis when given by daily injection (Figure 25).[105] Parathyroid hormone acts by stimulating bone turnover. Whilst bone resorption is increased, bone formation is stimulated to a greater degree, resulting in a marked anabolic effect. The treatment appears to be generally well tolerated, although hypercalcaemia has been recorded in some patients. Because of the need for regular injections, PTH treatment will probably be reserved for patients with severe osteoporosis who remain at high risk of fractures, even when treated with conventional agents.

Combination therapies

There are a number of published reports of using combination therapy in women with established osteoporosis. These include alendronate plus oestrogen, alendronate plus raloxifene, risedronate plus oestrogen, calcitonin plus oestrogen and PTH plus oestrogen. In general, combination therapy has resulted in slightly greater increases in BMD than were seen when either drug was used alone. However, these increments in BMD were not always statistically significant and there has been no documentation of any synergism when two drugs have been used in combination. Additionally, there are no fracture data to support the use of combination therapy.

Agents in development

Agents in development for the treatment of established osteoporosis include intravenous zoledronate, intravenous and oral ibandronate, and oral strontium ranelate. Zoledronate and ibandronate are potent bisphosphonates which have been shown to increase bone mass and inhibit bone resorption for prolonged periods after intravenous injection.[91, 92] Fracture data are awaited. Strontium ranelate substitutes for calcium in hydroxyapatite crystals and increases bone density. Fracture data are not yet available.

Corticosteroid-induced Osteoporosis

Corticosteroid treatment is an important cause of osteoporosis in patients with chronic inflammatory diseases and respiratory diseases. Population-based surveys have shown that approximately 0.5% of the UK population are taking long-term oral steroids and this figure increases to 1.7% in subjects aged 65 or over.[46] The risk of fragility fractures is increased 1.8-fold in asthmatic patients treated with oral corticosteroids when compared with non-steroid-treated asthmatics. Studies in patients with rheumatoid arthritis have also shown that corticosteroids increase fracture risk. Rheumatoid patients who have not received steroid treatment have a 2.1-fold increased risk of hip fracture when compared with controls and the risk increases to 2.7-fold in steroid-treated rheumatoid arthritis patients.[110] High-dose inhaled steroid therapy is also associated with reduced bone mass and it has been estimated that BMD falls by about 1% for each year patients have been taking 1000 mcg inhaled steroid daily.[111]

Pathogenesis

Several factors contribute to the pathogenesis of corticosteroid-induced osteoporosis.[47] Corticosteroids directly inhibit intestinal calcium absorption from the gut, probably by antagonizing the effects of 1,25-hydroxyvitamin D_3 on intestinal cells. They also cause an increase in urinary calcium losses by inhibiting calcium reabsorption by the renal tubules. The increased urinary losses of calcium, coupled with suppression of intestinal calcium absorption, causes serum calcium values to fall and PTH levels to rise. The raised levels of PTH stimulate bone turnover, but this is characterized by uncoupling of bone resorption from bone formation because corticosteroids inhibit bone formation by causing osteoblast apoptosis. The end result is accelerated bone loss, which is related to the dose and duration of corticosteroid therapy. Other factors which contribute to the pathogenesis of

steroid-induced osteoporosis include hypogonadism caused by suppression of the hypothalamic–pituitary axis in patients on high-dose steroids, and the adverse effects of underlying diseases such as rheumatoid arthritis and inflammatory bowel disease on bone mass.

Investigation

Patients who are thought to require more than 7.5 mg prednisolone daily for more than 3 months should undergo bone densitometry. If this shows a T-score of −1.5 or below then treatment is indicated. Even in subjects where the T-score is initially above −1.5, it is probably wise to repeat bone density at yearly intervals so long as the patient continues on steroids. Treatment should be considered if the BMD falls by more than 15% or if the T-score falls below −1.5. The reason for choosing a BMD T-score value of −1.5 as the threshold for intervention in steroid-induced osteoporosis is that the risk of fracture is extremely high in steroid-treated patients at levels of BMD which would not be associated with a significant increase in fracture risk in normal individuals. An illustration of this is provided by the studies of etidronate and risedronate therapy patients on steroid therapy. Even though the average BMD T-score value at baseline in these studies was only −1.5, approximately 25% of patients treated with calcium and vitamin D developed new vertebral fractures over the subsequent year.[112, 113]

Prevention and treatment

Since corticosteroids inhibit calcium absorption from the intestine by antagonizing the effects of vitamin D, calcium and vitamin D supplements should be given routinely to all patients, irrespective of the BMD value. This is supported by data from randomized clinical trials, which have shown that calcium and vitamin D supplements significantly inhibit bone loss in patients on low-dose steroids (<7.5 mg prednisolone daily).[114] Calcium and vitamin D do not prevent bone loss in steroid-treated patients, however, and have not been shown to prevent steroid-induced fractures.

Additional therapy is therefore required in patients with T-scores below –1.5 and/or a history of fracture. Several treatments are available, but bisphosphonates are probably the most effective agents. Cyclical etidronate has been found in several randomized controlled studies to increase BMD in corticosteroid-treated patients. In a meta-analysis of these studies,[115]Adachi *et al.* found that etidronate increased spine BMD by about 4% and hip BMD by about 1% when compared with standard therapy (either calcium, or calcium and vitamin D). Cyclical etidronate was found to significantly reduce the rate of new vertebral fractures in one study, but the effect was non-significant when data from all studies were combined (relative risk 0.50, 95% CI 0.21–1.19). Oral alendronate in doses of 5 and 10 mg daily has been found to increase BMD in patients at risk of corticosteroid-induced osteoporosis.[116] The average increase over 1 year was about 3% at the spine and 1% at the hip, compared with a fall of 0.5% and 1% at both sites in calcium-supplemented placebo. The rate of new vertebral fractures was 2.3% in alendronate-treated patients compared with 3.7%, but these differences were not significant due to the small number of events. The most convincing data on fracture prevention in patients with steroid-induced osteoporosis come from randomized placebo-controlled studies of risedronate. Two separate studies of risedronate (2.5 and 5 mg daily) combined with calcium and vitamin D have been conducted in patients with steroid-induced osteoporosis.[112, 117] A combined analysis of data from both studies showed that risedronate increased BMD by about 2% at the spine and 1% at the hip, whereas there was loss of bone in patients given calcium- and vitamin D-supplemented placebo. A significant reduction in the incidence of new vertebral fractures was noted in the 5 mg dose group when compared with placebo (Figure 26).

Other agents that have been studied in patients with steroid-induced osteoporosis include: HRT, calcitonin, and triple therapy with calcitriol, calcitonin and calcium. Hormone replacement therapy has not been shown to be effective in the prevention of steroid-induced bone loss or in preventing fractures associated with steroid therapy, but may be indicated

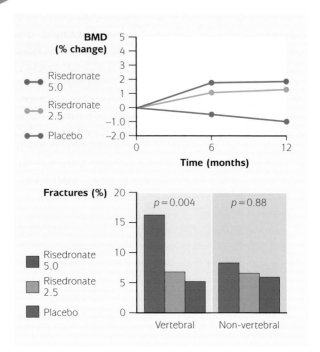

Figure 26. Effects of risedronate on BMD and fracture incidence in corticosteroid-induced osteoporosis. Adapted with permission from Wallach S *et al*. Effects of risedronate treatment on bone density and vertebral fracture in patients on corticosteroid therapy. *Calcif Tiss Int* 2000; **67**: 277–285.[112]

as an adjunct to other treatments in patients with clinical and biochemical evidence of hypogonadism. Calcitonin has been studied by several investigators in the prevention and treatment of steroid-induced osteoporosis. Whilst beneficial effects on BMD and fractures have been reported in a number of small, uncontrolled studies, randomized controlled studies have yielded mixed results. A small study published by Healey and colleagues showed no beneficial effect of calcitonin (100 IU) given by injection three times weekly on fracture or BMD in patients who were starting steroid medication for rheumatic diseases.[118] Both calcitonin and placebo groups also received calcium and vitamin D. In another study, Sambrook *et al.* randomized 103 patients starting steroid treatment to calcium (1000 mg daily), calcium plus calcitriol (0.5–1.0 mcg/day), or calcium plus calcitriol plus intranasal calcitonin (400 IU daily).[119] Both calcitriol groups slowed bone loss at the spine after 1 year when compared with calcium, but there was no effect on hip bone loss. After 2 years, bone loss remained significantly lower in the calcium plus calcitriol plus calcitonin group when compared with the calcium group, but had increased in the calcium plus calcitriol group, possibly because of an increase in steroid dose.

Osteoporosis in Men

The subject of osteoporosis in men has been neglected for many years, even though 30% of hip fractures and 20% of vertebral fractures occur in men. Secondary osteoporosis occurs frequently in men and accounts for up to 50% of cases of male osteoporosis seen in hospital practice (Figure 27).[120] The most common causes are hypogonadism, glucocorticoid use, alcoholism, neoplasia or a combination of these factors.[121] Other risk factors for low bone mass which have been identified by epidemiological surveys in men include low body weight, gastrectomy, hypertension, smoking, chronic chest disease and peptic ulcer disease.[122]

Pathogenesis

The pathogenesis of osteoporosis in men is less well understood than in women, but many risk factors are shared

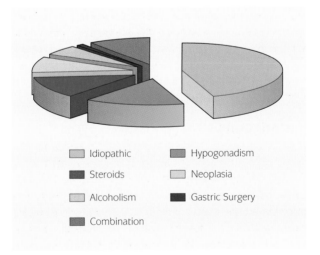

▦ Idiopathic		▦ Hypogonadism
▦ Steroids		▦ Neoplasia
▦ Alcoholism		▦ Gastric Surgery
▦ Combination		

Figure 27. Causes of osteoporosis in men with vertebral fractures. Data from Baillie SP *et al*. Pathogenesis of vertebral crush fractures in men. *Age Ageing* 1992; **21**: 139–141.[120]

in common. Sex hormones play an important role in regulating bone mass in men. Hypogonadism during skeletal growth is associated with low peak bone mass and increased bone loss during adulthood. Although androgens have traditionally been considered as the most important modulators of bone health in men, there is increasing evidence to suggest that the skeletal manifestations of androgen deficiency may be due to deficiency of oestrogen at the level of bone tissue, due to the conversion of androgens to oestrogen in peripheral tissues by aromatase.[123] Genetic factors also play an important role in the regulation of BMD in men. A positive family history of osteoporosis has been found to be associated with low bone mass in family studies,[124] and twin studies have suggested that the genetic contribution to fracture risk may be higher in men than in women.[125] The genes responsible for regulation of BMD and fracture risk in men have been relatively little researched. Candidate gene studies have identified allelic associations between BMD and/or osteoporotic fracture in men, and polymorphisms of the VDR gene, COLIA1 gene, ER-α gene and aromatase gene.[126] Inactivating mutations of the ER-α and aromatase genes have been described in association with osteoporosis in males, although this is extremely rare. Whilst some of the genes responsible for susceptibility to osteoporosis in men and women overlap, linkage studies in mice indicate that there may be some genes which are specific to the regulation of BMD in men.[127]

Investigation

Bone densitometry is the investigation of choice for the diagnosis of male osteoporosis, although the BMD T-score values at which treatment should be started are less well defined than in women. Low BMD values predispose to osteoporotic fractures in men, and epidemiological studies have shown that the absolute risk of fracture is the same in men and women for any given level of BMD. It has been suggested that the female T-score cut-off of −2.5 may be inappropriate for the diagnosis of osteoporosis in men, and that a threshold of −2.0 may be better, since it more accurately

Table 13. Investigation for secondary causes of osteoporosis in men

Routine biochemical and haematological screen:
- Assessment of thyroid function
- Liver function tests
- Assessment of calcium biochemistry
- Assessment of serum proteins

Full blood count

ESR

Immunoglobulins

Serum testosterone

Gonadotrophins

Other endocrine investigations if pituitary or adrenal disorders are suspected

reflects the prevalence of osteoporotic fractures in men.[128] Investigation for secondary causes of osteoporosis is particularly important, since these are common in males with osteoporosis (Table 13). A routine biochemical and haematological screen, including assessment of thyroid function, liver function tests, calcium biochemistry and serum proteins, should be performed. Full blood count, ESR and immunoglobulins should be performed to screen for inflammatory disease and myeloma. Serum testosterone and gonadotrophins should be checked in all patients. Other endocrine investigations may be required in some cases if there is clinical suspicion of a pituitary or adrenal disorder.

Treatment

Patients should be advised against smoking and taking alcohol in excess. Exercise should be encouraged. Underlying diseases should be treated where possible, and calcium and vitamin D supplementation given when dietary intake is suboptimal. Androgen replacement with testosterone should be given to hypogonadal patients, although it is unclear if androgens are of benefit in the treatment of eugonadal men with osteoporosis. Uncontrolled short-term studies have shown that injections of testosterone in doses of 250 mg per month increase BMD and suppress biochemical markers of bone turnover in eugonadal osteoporotic men, but the long-term safety and efficacy of this treatment has not been established.[129] Treatment with the bisphosphonate alendronate has been shown to increase bone mass and reduce the incidence of new vertebral fractures in men with osteoporosis. The pivotal study is that of Orwoll *et al.*, who randomized 241 men with osteoporosis to receive alendronate (10 mg daily) or a matching placebo for 2 years, along with calcium and vitamin D supplements.[130] The patients were selected on the basis that they had previous vertebral fractures (present in 50% of the study group) or had low BMD values (femoral neck T-score less than –2.0 and lumbar spine T-score less that –1). Alendronate increased spine BMD by about 5% and femoral neck BMD by about 2.5% when compared with placebo, reduced bone turnover, stopped height loss and significantly reduced the incidence of new morphometrically defined vertebral fractures from 7% to 0.8%.

There is limited information on the use of other bisphosphonates such as risedronate and etidronate in men with osteoporosis, although the therapeutic effect of these agents in men with steroid-induced osteoporosis seems to be equivalent to that in women with steroid-induced osteoporosis. Cyclical sodium fluoride in low doses (15 mg daily given 3 months on, 1 month off) plus calcium supplements were found to increase spine BMD and reduce the incidence of new vertebral fractures in one study of male osteoporotic patients, when compared with calcium alone, although the study was not blinded.[131] Pilot studies have also been performed in which fluoride has been combined with etidronate in men with osteoporosis. These studies have shown a greater effect of combined therapy on BMD, but the effects on fracture incidence are unknown. There is no information on the effects of calcitonin, raloxifene, tibolone or active vitamin D metabolites in the treatment of osteoporosis in men.

Osteogenesis Imperfecta

Pathogenesis

Osteogenesis imperfecta (OI) is a rare inherited bone disease, which is characterized by increased bone fragility and multiple fractures. Most cases of OI are caused by mutations in the COLIA1 and COLIA2 genes, which encode the α1 and α2 chains of type I collagen,[132] although other subtypes have recently been described which are unlinked to the collagen genes.[133, 134] Osteogenesis imperfecta is usually inherited in an autosomal dominant fashion, although a positive family history is not always found, since many cases are new mutations. A large number of mutations have been described which cause OI, and the clinical picture depends on the nature and site of the mutation (Table 14).

Non-sense and mis-sense mutations affecting the triple helical domain of the collagen molecule typically cause severe OI, which can be neonatal lethal (type II) or be associated with severe skeletal deformity because of multiple fractures in infancy (type III). Bone fragility is less marked in osteogenesis imperfecta types I and IV. Type I OI is characterized by blue sclerae (Figure 28) and is most commonly caused by splice site mutations in the COLIA1 gene. This results in degradation of RNA derived from the mutant allele and results in the reduced production of structurally normal COLIA1 protein chains. Type IV OI can be caused by mutations affecting the coding regions of COLIA1 or COLIA2. These mutations alter the protein sequence, but bone fragility is less severe than in type II and III OI, presumably because the amino acid substitution has less effect on the stability of the collagen molecule. Rarely, conservative mutations in the collagen type I genes occur, resulting in a syndrome of increased bone fragility and reduced bone mass, which resembles severe osteoporosis. Examination of bone tissue in patients with OI has revealed several abnormalities of bone turnover and bone

Table 14. Clinical classification of osteogenesis imperfecta

Type	Phenotype	Clinical features	Mutations
I	Mild, non-deforming	Blue sclerae. Dental abnormalities in some cases. Hearing loss	Null allele COLIA1. Conservative protein coding mutations in COLIA1 and COLIA2
II	Lethal	Extreme bone fragility	Coding mutations in COLIA1/COLIA2
III	Severe, deforming	Normal sclerae. Short stature	Coding mutations in COLIA1/COLIA2
IV	Moderate, sometimes deforming	Normal sclerae. Dental abnormalities in some cases	Coding mutations in COLIA1/COLIA2
V	Severe, deforming	Hypertrophic callus around fractures	Gene unknown
VI	Moderate, sometimes deforming	Sclerae white or slightly blue. Defective mineralization of bone	Gene unknown

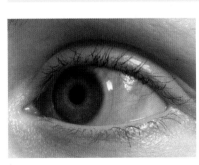

Figure 28. Blue sclerae in type I OI.

mineralization. The rate of bone turnover is increased in OI and woven bone may be observed on histological examination.

Why this should happen is poorly understood, but it has been suggested that the presence of abnormal collagen chains may act as a stimulus to bone turnover. Mineralization of the bone is also abnormally increased.[135] This has been attributed to the fact that collagen fibrils are arranged abnormally, allowing hydroxyapatite crystals to be deposited at a greater density than is usual. The very high levels of mineralization observed in OI are thought to increase bone fragility by increasing the brittleness of bone tissue.

Investigation and diagnosis

The diagnosis of OI should be suspected in children with a history of recurrent fractures on minimal trauma. Child abuse and idiopathic juvenile osteoporosis are the commonest differential diagnoses. In some cases, typical clinical features of OI such as blue sclera and abnormal dentition may be observed, but these abnormalities are not seen in all patients. Radiological examination of the skull may reveal wormian bones, but this is not diagnostic. Bone density is often reduced in OI, but not invariably so, and this investigation is not useful in distinguishing OI from idiopathic juvenile osteoporosis. The diagnosis of OI can be made by examining the relative abundance of $\alpha 1$ and $\alpha 2$ collagen chains produced by cultured skin fibroblasts (type I) or the thermal stability of collagen protein chains (types II–IV) produced by cultured skin fibroblasts. The diagnosis can also be made by sequencing of the collagen cDNA, although this does not detect type I OI.

Management

The management of OI is difficult, in view of the fact that the underlying problem is a fundamental abnormality in collagen abundance and/or structure. Prompted by the observation that bone turnover is increased, several investigators have used bone resorption inhibitors in the treatment of OI and most interest has focused on the use of intravenous pamidronate. The most comprehensive study is that of Glorieux and colleagues,[136] who administered cyclical intravenous pamidronate (three infusions of 1.5–3.0 mg/kg every 3 months) to a series of 30 children with severe OI and multiple fractures. The treatment causes a reduction in bone pain, a dramatic reduction in the rate of new bone fractures, a decrease in bone turnover markers, an increase in the size of vertebral bodies and an increase in BMD. Placebo-controlled studies are now in progress to look at the effects of oral bisphosphonate therapy in patients with OI. Women with OI should be treated with HRT or bisphosphonate therapy at the time of menopause to prevent bone loss associated with oestrogen deficiency, in the light of data which have shown a dramatic increase in fracture rates after the menopause.[137]

Other Rare Causes of Osteoporosis

Idiopathic juvenile osteoporosis presents at the age of 8–12 years with fractures, bone pain or kyphosis, without the stigmata or family history of OI.[138] The cause of this condition is unclear and there is no consensus with regard to the best mode of treatment. Intravenous pamidronate has been used in some cases, and was found to improve bone pain and increase BMD.[139] Osteoporosis can also present in pregnancy with vertebral fractures and kyphosis, when it is referred to as pregnancy-associated osteoporosis.[140] It is currently unclear if this is a specific entity or a manifestation of the physiological bone loss during pregnancy in patients who have pre-existing osteoporosis. It is unclear how these patients should best be treated. Bisphosphonates and other anti-osteoporosis drugs are contraindicated during pregnancy because of the potential adverse effects on the foetus. Calcium and vitamin D supplements are often given empirically, but it is unclear whether or not they have any effect on the natural history of the disease. Osteoporosis can occur in haematological diseases such as sickle cell anaemia and thallasaemia, and in infiltrative disorders of bone marrow such as Gaucher's disease and systemic mastocytosis. The pathogenesis of osteoporosis in these conditions is unclear and there is little information on how bone loss in these conditions should be treated.

Frequently Asked Questions

What is osteoporosis?
Osteoporosis is a disease caused by thinning of the bones. This leads to increased bone fragility and increases the risk of a bone fracture occurring.

Am I at risk of osteoporosis?
Osteoporosis mainly affects women after the menopause. Only 1–2% of women under the age of about 40 have osteoporosis, but the prevalence increases to affect about 15% of women by the age of 60 and 40% of women by the age of 80.

Can men get osteoporosis?
Osteoporosis is less common in men. Between 1% and 2% of men under 40 have osteoporosis, but the prevalence increases to 7% by the age of 65 and 16% by the age of 80.

What causes osteoporosis?
Many risk factors have been identified, including poor diet, lack of exercise, smoking, low body weight and corticosteroid treatment. Genetic factors play an important role and a positive family history is an important risk factor.

Does osteoporosis cause symptoms?
Thinning of the bones does not cause symptoms on its own, but symptoms such as back pain can develop when osteoporotic fractures occur.

How can I find out if I have osteoporosis?
Osteoporosis can be diagnosed by bone mineral density (BMD) scan. This should be performed if you have risk factors for osteoporosis such as a positive family history or early menopause.

Can osteoporosis be prevented or treated?

Several treatments are available to prevent osteoporosis and fractures caused by osteoporosis. These treatments may be required if you are found to have low bone density or have suffered a fragility fracture.

What is a fragility fracture?

Fragility fractures are fractures that occur for no reason, or as the result of a fall from standing height or less.

Should I be on a special diet?

It is important that your diet contains enough calcium and vitamin D. Dairy products such as milk, cheese and yoghurt are the main sources of calcium in the diet. Men should take the equivalent of 1 pint of milk per day and women 1.5 pints per day to maintain bone health. Skimmed milk and low fat milk products contain the same amount of calcium as full cream milk.

What about alcohol?

Moderate alcohol intake (<20 units per week for women and <30 units per week for men) does not increase the risk of osteoporosis and if anything it may be protective. Levels of alcohol intake above these are detrimental for the skeleton and can lead to osteoporosis.

What about smoking?

Smoking increases the risk of osteoporosis and bone fractures. There are many reasons for this; important ones include the fact that smokers have an earlier menopause than non-smokers, take less exercise and tend to have low body weight.

Do I need to give up any sports or hobbies?

You should be able to continue most sporting and leisure activities as normal. In fact, physical activity is beneficial for sufferers of osteoporosis, since it seems to protect against bone loss and improves muscle strength, which reduces the risk of falling. The only thing to avoid is lifting heavy weights or straining your back, since this can cause spine fractures.

Are my children and grandchildren at risk of osteoporosis?

The risk of osteoporosis is increased in children and other relatives of osteoporosis sufferers, although the disease is not inherited in a predictable way.

Can anything be done to prevent my children developing osteoporosis?

The risk of developing osteoporosis can be reduced if growing children take a good diet with plenty of calcium and if they take plenty of exercise.

Should my children have a bone density scan?

Bone density scans in children and young adults are not usually helpful in assessing the risk of osteoporosis. If there is a concern because of a family history of osteoporosis, bone scans are best performed around the age of 50, when bone loss starts to occur.

References

1. Cooper C, Melton LJ. Epidemiology of osteoporosis. *Trends Endocrinol Metab* 1992; **3**: 224–229.

2. Kanis JA, Melton LJ, Christiansen C *et al*. The diagnosis of osteoporosis. *J Bone Miner Res* 1994; **9**: 1137–1141.

3. Melton LJ. How many women have osteoporosis now? [Review]. *J Bone Miner Res* 1995; **10**: 175–177.

4. De Laet CE, van Hout BA, Burger H *et al*. Bone density and risk of hip fracture in men and women: cross sectional analysis. *Br Med J* 1997; **315**: 221–225 [published erratum appears in *Br Med J* 1997; **315**: 916].

5. Dargent-Molina P, Favier F, Grandjean H *et al*. Fall-related factors and risk of hip fracture: the EPIDOS prospective study. Epidemiologie de l'osteoporose. *Lancet* 1996; **348**: 145–149.

6. Cummings SR, Kelsey JL, Nevitt MC, O'Dowd KJ. Epidemiology of osteoporosis and osteoporotic fractures. *Epidemiol Rev* 1985; **7**: 178–208.

7. Cummings SR, Cauley JA, Palermo L *et al*. Racial differences in hip axis lengths might explain racial differences in rates of hip fracture. Study of Osteoporotic Fractures Research Group. *Osteoporosis Int* 1994; **4**: 226–229.

8. Balemans W, Ebeling M, Patel N *et al*. Increased bone density in sclerosteosis is due to the deficiency of a novel secreted protein (SOST). *Hum Molec Genet* 2001; **10**: 537–543.

9. Ducy P, Schinke T, Karsenty G. The osteoblast: a sophisticated fibroblast under central surveillance. *Science* 2000; **289**: 1501–1504.

10. Nakashima K, Zhou X, Kunkel G *et al*. The novel zinc finger-containing transcription factor osterix is required for osteoblast differentiation and bone formation. *Cell* 2002; **108**: 17–29.

11. Noble BS, Reeve J. Osteocyte function, osteocyte death and bone fracture resistance. *Molec Cell Endocrinol* 2000; **159**: 7–13.

12. Everts V, Delaisse JM, Korper W *et al*. The bone lining cell: its role in cleaning Howship's lacunae and initiating bone formation. *J Bone Miner Res* 2002; **17**: 77–90.

13. Teitelbaum SL. Bone resorption by osteoclasts. *Science* 2000; **289**: 1504–1508.

14. Sykes B, Smith R. Collagen and collagen gene disorders. *Quart J Med* 1985; **221**: 533–547.

15. Knott L, Bailey AJ. Collagen cross-links in mineralizing tissues: a review of their chemistry, function, and clinical relevance. *Bone* 1998; **22**: 181–187.

16. Raisz LG. Physiology and pathophysiology of bone remodeling. *Clin Chem* 1999; **45**: 1353–1358 [published erratum appears in *Clin Chem* 1999; **45**: 1885].

17. Stewart TL, Ralston SH. Role of genetic factors in the pathogenesis of osteoporosis. *J Endocrinol* 2000; **166**: 235–245.

18. Arden NK, Baker J, Hogg C *et al*. The heritability of bone mineral density, ultrasound of the calcaneus and hip axis length: a study of postmenopausal twins. *J Bone Miner Res* 1996; **11**: 530–534.

19. Hunter D, de Lange M, Snieder H *et al*. Genetic contribution to bone metabolism, calcium excretion, and vitamin D and parathyroid hormone regulation. *J Bone Miner Res* 2001; **16**: 371–378.

20. Torgerson DJ, Campbell MK, Thomas RE, Reid DM. Prediction of perimenopausal fractures by bone mineral density and other risk factors. *J Bone Miner Res* 1996; **11**: 293–297.

21. Gong Y, Slee RB, Fukai N *et al*. LDL receptor-related protein 5 (LRP5) affects bone accrual and eye development. *Cell* 2001; **107**: 513–523.

22. Eisman JA. Genetics of osteoporosis. *Endocrinol Rev* 1999; **20**: 788–804.

23. Becherini L, Gennari L, Masi L *et al*. Evidence of a linkage disequilibrium between polymorphisms in the human estrogen receptor alpha gene and their relationship to bone mass variation in postmenopausal Italian women. *Hum Molec Genet* 2000; **9**: 2043–2050.

24. Masi L, Becherini L, Gennari L *et al*. Polymorphism of the aromatase gene in postmenopausal Italian women: distribution and correlation with bone mass and fracture risk. *J Clin Endocrinol Metab* 2001; **86**: 2263–2269.

25. Mann V, Hobson EE, Li B *et al*. A COLIA1 Sp1 binding site polymorphism predisposes to osteoporotic fracture by affecting bone density and quality. *J Clin Invest* 2001; **107**: 899–907.

26. Yamada Y, Miyauchi A, Takagi Y *et al*. Association of the C-509T polymorphism, alone or in combination with the T869C polymorphism, or the transforming growth factor-beta1 gene with bone mineral density and genetic susceptibility to osteoporosis in Japanese women. *J Molec Med* 2001; **79**: 149–156.

27. Janssens K, Gershoni-Baruch R, Guanabens N *et al*. Mutations in the gene encoding the latency-associated peptide of TGF-beta1 cause Camurati–Engelmann disease. *Nat Genet* 2000; **26**: 273–275.

28. Little RD, Carulli JP, Del Mastro RG *et al*. A mutation in the LDL receptor-related protein 5 gene results in the autosomal dominant high-bone-mass trait. *Am J Hum Genet* 2002; **70**: 11–19.

29. Pacifici R. Estrogen, cytokines, and pathogenesis of postmenopausal osteoporosis. *J Bone Miner Res* 1996; **11**: 1043–1051.

30. Riggs BL, Khosla S, Melton LJ. Sex steroids and the construction and conservation of the adult skeleton. *J Cell Biochem* 2002; **23**: 279–302.

31. Reid DM, New SA. Nutritional influences on bone mass. *Proc Nutr Soc* 1997; **56**: 977–987.

32. Murphy S, Khaw KT, May H, Compston JE. Milk consumption and bone mineral density in middle aged and elderly women. *Br Med J* 1994; **308**: 939–941.

33. Reid IR, Ames RW, Evans M *et al*. Effect of calcium supplementation on bone loss in postmenopausal women. *New Engl J Med* 1993; **328**: 460–464.

34. Riggotti NA, Nussbaum SR, Hertzog DB *et al*. Osteoporosis in women with anorexia nervosa. *New Engl J Med* 1984; **311**: 1601–1606.

35. Skerry TM. Mechanical loading and bone: what sort of exercise is beneficial to the skeleton? *Bone* 1997; **20**: 179–181.

36. Drinkwater BL, Nilson K, Chestnut CH *et al*. Bone mineral content of amenorrheic and eumenorrheic athletes. *New Engl J Med* 1984; **311**: 277–281.

37. Law MR, Hackshaw AK. A meta-analysis of cigarette smoking, bone mineral density and risk of hip fracture: recognition of a major effect. *Br Med J* 1997; **315**: 841–846.

38. Feitelberg S, Epstein S, Ismail F, D'Amanda C. Deranged bone mineral metabolism in chronic alcoholism. *Metabolism* 1987; **36**: 322–326.

39. Black AJ, Topping J, Durham B *et al*. A detailed assessment of alterations in bone turnover, calcium homeostasis, and bone density in normal pregnancy. *J Bone Miner Res* 2000; **15**: 557–563.

40. Croucher PI, Vedi S, Motley RJ *et al*. Reduced bone formation in patients with osteoporosis associated with inflammatory bowel disease. *Osteoporosis Int* 1993; **3**: 236–241.

41. Reid DM, Harvie J. Secondary osteoporosis. *Baillieres Clin Endocrinol Metab* 1997; **11**: 83–99.

42. Mora S, Barera G, Ricotti A *et al*. Reversal of low bone density with a gluten-free diet in children and adolescents with celiac disease. *Am J Clin Nutr* 1998; **67**: 477–481.

43. Paul TL, Kerrigan J, Kelly AM *et al*. Long-term L-thyroxine therapy is associated with decreased hip bone density in premenopausal women. *J Am Med Assoc* 1988; **259**: 3137–3141.

44. Cummings SR, Nevitt MC, Browner WS *et al*. Risk factors for hip fracture in white women. Study of Osteoporotic Fractures Research Group. *New Engl J Med* 1995; **332**: 767–773.

45. Silverberg SJ, Shane E, Jacobs TP *et al*. A 10-year prospective study of primary hyperparathyroidism with or without parathyroid surgery. *New Engl J Med* 1999; **341**: 1249–1255.

46. Walsh LJ, Wong CA, Pringle M *et al*. Use of oral corticosteroids in the community and the prevention of secondary osteoporosis: a cross sectional study. *Br Med J* 1996; **313**: 344–346.

47. Reid IR, Grey AB. Corticosteroid osteoporosis. In: Reid DM, editor. *Bailliere's Clinical Rheumatology*. London: Bailliere Tindall, 1993; pp. 573–587.

48. Oefelein MG, Ricchuiti V, Conrad W *et al*. Skeletal fracture associated with androgen suppression induced osteoporosis: the

clinical incidence and risk factors for patients with prostate cancer. *J Urol* 2001; **166**: 1724–1728.

49. Cummings SR, Black DM, Nevitt MC *et al*. Bone density at various sites for prediction of hip fractures. The Study of Osteoporotic Fractures Research Group. *Lancet* 1993; **341**: 72–75.

50. Siris ES, Miller PD, Barrett-Connor E *et al*. Identification and fracture outcomes of undiagnosed low bone mineral density in postmenopausal women: results from the National Osteoporosis Risk Assessment. *J Am Med Assoc* 2001; **286**: 2815–2822.

51. Bauer DC, Gluer CC, Genent HK, Stone K. Quantitative ultrasound and vertebral fracture in postmenapausal women. Fracture Intervention Trial Research Group. *J Bone Miner Res* 1995; **10**: 353–358.

52. Ahmed AI, Ilic D, Blake G, *et al*. Review of 3,530 referrals for bone density measurements of spine and femur: evidence that radiographic osteopenia predicts low bone mass. *Radiology* 1998; **207**: 619–624.

53. Ismail AA, Cooper C, Felsenberg D *et al*. Number and type of vertebral deformities: epidemiological characteristics and relation to back pain and height loss. European Vertebral Osteoporosis Study Group. *Osteoporosis Int* 1999; **9**: 206–213.

54. Garrero P, Hausherr E, Chapuy MC *et al*. Markers of bone resorption predict hip fracture in elderly women: the EPIDOS study. *J Bone Miner Res* 1996; **11**: 1531–1538.

55. Dawson-Hughes B, Dallal G, Krall E *et al*. A controlled trial of the effect of calcium supplements on bone density in post-menopausal women. *New Engl J Med* 1990; **323**: 878–883.

56. Bonjour J-P, Carrie AL, Ferrari S *et al*. Calcium-enriched foods and bone mass growth in prepubertal girls: a randomized, double-blind, placebo-controlled trial. *J Clin Invest* 1997; **99**: 1287–1294

57. Cleghorn DB, O'Loughlin PD, Schroeder BJ, Nordin BE. An open, crossover trial of calcium-fortified milk in prevention of early postmenopausal bone loss. *Med J Aust* 2001; **175**: 242–245.

58. Wallace BA, Cumming RG. Systematic review of randomized trials of the effect of exercise on bone mass in pre- and postmenopausal women. *Calcif Tiss Int* 2000; **67**: 10–18.

59. Lau E, Donnan S, Barker DJP, Cooper C. Physical activity and calcium intake in fracture of the proximal femur in Hong Kong. *Br Med J* 1988; **297**: 1441–1443.

60. Welten DC, Kemper HC, Post GB *et al*. Weight-bearing activity during youth is a more important factor for peak bone mass than calcium intake. *J Bone Miner Res* 1994; **9**: 1089–1096.

61. Reid IR, Ames RW, Evans MC *et al*. Long-term effects of calcium supplementation on bone loss and fractures in postmenopausal women: a randomized controlled trial. *Am J Med* 1995; **98**: 331–335.

62. Krall EA, Parry P, Lichter JB, Dawson-Hughes B. Vitamin D receptor alleles and rates of bone loss: influence of years since menopause and calcium intake. *J Bone Miner Res* 1995; **10**: 978–984.

63. Lips P, Graafmans WC, Ooms ME *et al*. Vitamin D supplementation and fracture incidence in elderly persons. A randomized, placebo-controlled clinical trial. *Ann Intern Med* 1996; **124**: 400–406.

64. Ooms ME, Roos JC, Bezemer PD *et al*. Prevention of bone loss by vitamin D supplementation in elderly women: a randomized double-blind trial. *J Clin Endocrinol Metab* 1995; **80**: 1052–1058.

65. Graafmans WC, Lips P, Ooms ME *et al*. The effect of Vitamin D supplementation on the bone mineral density of the femoral neck is associated with vitamin D receptor genotype. *J Bone Miner Res* 1997; **12**: 1241–1245.

66. Dawson-Hughes B, Harris SS, Krall EA, Dallal GE. Effect of calcium and vitamin D supplementation on bone density in men and women 65 years of age or older. *New Engl J Med* 1997; **337**: 670–676.

67. Chapuy MC, Arlot ME, Delmas PD, Meunier PJ. Effect of calcium and cholecalciferol treatment for three years on hip fractures in elderly women. *Br Med J* 1994; **308**: 1081–1082.

68. Chapuy MC, Arlot ME, Duboeuf F *et al*. Vitamin D3 and calcium to prevent hip fractures in the elderly women. *New Engl J Med* 1992; **327**: 1637–1642.

69. Torgerson DJ, Bell-Syer SE. Hormone replacement therapy and prevention of nonvertebral fractures: a meta-analysis of randomized trials. *J Am Med Assoc* 2001; **285**: 2891–2897.

70. Lufkin EG, Wahner HW, O'Fallon WM *et al*. Treatment of postmenopausal osteoporosis with transdermal estrogen. *Ann Intern Med* 1992; **117**: 1–9.

71. Lindsay R, Hart DM, Forrest C, Baird C. Prevention of spinal osteoporosis in oophorectomised women. *Lancet* 1980; **ii**: 1151–1154.

72. Gallacher JC, Riggs BL, DeLuca HF. Effect of estrogen on calcium absorption and serum vitamin D metabolites in post-menopausal osteoporosis. *J Clin Endocrinol Metab* 1980; **51**: 1359–1364.

73. Collaborative Group on Hormonal Factors in Breast Cancer. Breast cancer and hormone replacement therapy: collaborative reanalysis of data from 51 epidemiological studies of 52,705 women with breast cancer and 108,411 women without breast cancer. *Lancet* 1997; **350**: 1047–1059.

74. Writing Group for the Women's Health Initiative Investigators. Risks and benefits of estrogen plus progestin in healthy postmenopausal women: principal results from the Women's Health Initiative randomized controlled trial. *J Am Med Assoc* 2002; **288**: 321–333.

75. Hulley S, Grady D, Bush T *et al*. Randomized trial of estrogen plus progestin for secondary prevention of coronary heart disease in postmenopausal women. Heart and Estrogen/progestin Replacement Study (HERS) Research Group. *J Am Med Assoc* 1998; **280**: 605–613.

76. Cauley JA, Seeley DG, Ensrud K *et al*. Estrogen replacement therapy and fractures in older women. Study of Osteoporotic Fractures Research Group. *Ann Intern Med* 1995; **122**: 9–16.

77. Delmas PD, Bjarnason NH, Mitlak BH *et al*. Effects of raloxifene on bone mineral density, serum cholesterol concentrations, and uterine endometrium in post-menopausal women. *New Engl J Med* 1997; **337**: 1641–1647.

78. Ettinger B, Black DM, Mitlak BH *et al*. Reduction of vertebral fracture risk in postmenopausal women with osteoporosis treated with raloxifene. *J Am Med Assoc* 1999; **282**: 637–645.

79. Cummings SR, Eckert S, Krueger KA *et al*. The effect of raloxifene on risk of breast cancer in postmenopausal women:

results from the MORE randomized trial. Multiple Outcomes of Raloxifene Evaluation. *J Am Med Assoc* 1999; **281**: 2189–2197.

80. Bjarnason NH, Bjarnason K, Haarbo J *et al*. Tibolone: prevention of bone loss in late postmenopausal women. *J Clin Endocrinol Metab* 1996; **81**: 2419–2422.

81. Hammar M, Christau S, Nathorst-Boos J *et al*. A double-blind, randomised trial comparing the effects of tibolone and continuous combined hormone replacement therapy in postmenopausal women with menopausal symptoms. *Br J Obstet Gynaecol* 1998; **105**: 904–911.

82. Herd RJ, Balena R, Blake GM *et al*. The prevention of early postmenopausal bone loss by cyclical etidronate therapy: a 2-year, double-blind, placebo-controlled study. *Am J Med* 1997; **103**: 92–99.

83. Hosking D, Chilvers CE, Christiansen C *et al*. Prevention of bone loss with alendronate in postmenopausal women under 60 years of age. Early Postmenopausal Intervention Cohort Study Group. *New Engl J Med* 1998; **338**: 485–492.

84. Liberman UA, Weiss SR, Broll J *et al*. Effect of oral alendronate on bone mineral density and the incidence of fractures in postmenopausal osteoporosis. The Alendronate Phase III Osteoporosis Treatment Study Group. *New Engl J Med* 1995; **333**: 1437–1443.

85. Cummings SR, Black DM, Thompson DE *et al*. Effect of alendronate on risk of fracture in women with low bone density but without vertebral fractures: results from the Fracture Intervention Trial. *J Am Med Assoc* 1998; **280**: 2077–2082.

86. Pols HA, Felsenberg D, Hanley DA *et al*. Multinational, placebo-controlled, randomized trial of the effects of alendronate on bone density and fracture risk in postmenopausal women with low bone mass: results of the FOSIT study. Fosamax International Trial Study Group. *Osteoporosis Int* 1999; **9**: 461–468.

87. Schnitzer T, Bone HG, Crepaldi G *et al*. Therapeutic equivalence of alendronate 70 mg once-weekly and alendronate 10 mg daily in the treatment of osteoporosis. Alendronate Once-Weekly Study Group. *Aging (Milano)* 2000; **12**: 1–12.

88. Kelly R, Taggart H. Incidence of gastrointestinal side effects due to alendronate is high in clinical practice. *Br Med J* 1997; **315**: 1235.

89. Fogelman I, Ribot C, Smith R *et al*. Risedronate reverses bone loss in postmenopausal women with low bone mass: results from a multinational, double-blind, placebo-controlled trial. BMD-MN Study Group. *J Clin Endocrinol Metab* 2000; **85**: 1895–1900.

90. McClung MR, Guesens P, Miller PD *et al*. Effect of risedronate on the risk of hip fracture in elderly women. *New Engl J Med* 2001; **344**: 333–340.

91. Reid IR, Brown JP, Burckhardt P *et al*. Intravenous zoledronic acid in postmenopausal women with low bone mineral density. *New Engl J Med* 2002; **346**: 653–661.

92. Thiebaud D, Burckhardt P, Kriegbaum H *et al*. Three monthly intravenous injections of ibandronate in the treatment of postmenopausal osteoporosis. *Am J Med* 1997; **103**: 298–307.

93. Eastell R, Reid DM, Compston J *et al*. Secondary prevention of osteoporosis: when should a non-vertebral fracture be a trigger for action? *Quart J Med* 2001; **94**: 575–597.

94. Lindsay R, Silverman SL, Cooper C *et al*. Risk of new vertebral fracture in the year following a fracture. *J Am Med Assoc* 2001; **285**: 320–323.

95. Ott SM, Chestnut CH. Calcitriol treatment is not effective in postmenopausal osteoporosis. *Ann Intern Med* 1989; **110**: 267–274.

96. Tilyard MW, Spears GF, Thomson J, Dovey S. Treatment of postmenopausal osteoporosis with calcitriol or calcium. *New Engl J Med* 1992; **326**: 357–362.

97. Orimo H, Shiraki M, Hayashi Y *et al*. Effects of 1 alpha-hydroxyvitamin D3 on lumbar bone mineral density and vertebral fractures in patients with postmenopausal osteoporosis. *Calcif Tiss Int* 1994; **54**: 370–376.

98. Chesnut CH, Silverman S, Andriano K *et al*. A randomized trial of nasal spray salmon calcitonin in postmenopausal women with established osteoporosis: the prevent recurrence of osteoporotic fractures study. *Am J Med* 2000; **109**: 267–276.

99. Haguenauer D, Welch V, Shea B *et al*. Fluoride for the treatment of postmenopausal osteoporotic fractures: a meta-analysis. *Osteoporosis Int* 2000; **11**: 727–738.

100. Storm T, Thamsborg G, Steiniche T *et al*. Effect of intermittent cyclical etidronate therapy on bone mass and fracture

rate in women with postmenopausal osteoporosis. *New Engl J Med* 1990; **322**: 1265–1271.

101. Watts NB, Harris ST, Genant HK *et al*. Intermittent cyclical etidronate treatment of postmenopausal osteoporosis. *New Engl J Med* 1990; **323**: 73–79.

102. van Staa TP, Abenhaim L, Cooper C. Use of cyclical etidronate and prevention of non-vertebral fractures. *Br J Rheumatol* 1998; **37**: 87–94.

103. Reginster J, Minne HW, Sorensen OH *et al*. Randomized trial of the effects of risedronate on vertebral fractures in women with established postmenopausal osteoporosis. Vertebral Efficacy with Risedronate Therapy (VERT) Study Group. *Osteoporosis Int* 2000; **11**: 83–91.

104. Harris ST, Watts NB, Genant HK *et al*. Effects of risedronate treatment on vertebral and nonvertebral fractures in women with postmenopausal osteoporosis: a randomized controlled trial. Vertebral Efficacy With Risedronate Therapy (VERT) Study Group. *J Am Med Assoc* 1999; **282**: 1344–1352

105. Neer RM, Arnaud CD, Zanchetta JR *et al*. Effect of parathyroid hormone (1–34) on fractures and bone mineral density in postmenopausal women with osteoporosis. *New Engl J Med* 2001; **344**: 1434–1441.

106. Kanis JA, McCloskey EV. Effect of calcitonin on vertebral and other fractures. *Quart J Med* 1999; **92**: 143–149.

107. Lyritis GP, Paspati I, Karachalios T *et al*. Pain relief from nasal salmon calcitonin in osteoporotic vertebral crush fractures. A double blind, placebo-controlled clinical study. *Acta Orthop Scand Suppl* 1997; **275**: 112–114.

108. Caverzasio J, Palmer G, Bonjour JP. Fluoride: mode of action. *Bone* 1998; **22**: 585–589.

109. Black DM, Cummings SR, Karpf DB *et al*. Randomised trial of effect of alendronate on risk of fracture in women with existing vertebral fractures. Fracture Intervention Trial Research Group. *Lancet* 1996; **348**: 1535–1541.

110. Cooper C, Coupland C, Mitchell M. Rheumatoid arthritis, corticosteroid therapy and hip fracture. *Ann Rheum Dis* 1995; **54**: 49–52.

111. Wong CA, Walsh LJ, Smith CJ *et al*. Inhaled corticosteroid use and bone-mineral density in patients with asthma. *Lancet* 2000; **355**: 1399–1403.

112. Wallach S, Cohen S, Reid DM *et al*. Effects of risedronate treatment on bone density and vertebral fracture in patients on corticosteroid therapy. *Calcif Tiss Int* 2000; **67**: 277–285.

113. Adachi JD, Bensen WG, Brown J *et al*. Intermittent etidronate therapy to prevent corticosteroid-induced osteoporosis. *New Engl J Med* 1997; **337**: 382–387.

114. Adachi JD, Bensen WG, Bianchi F *et al*. Vitamin D and calcium in the prevention of corticosteroid induced osteoporosis: a 3 year follow up. *J Rheumatol* 1996; **23**: 995–1000.

115. Adachi JD, Roux C, Pitt PI *et al*. A pooled data analysis on the use of intermittent cyclical etidronate therapy for the prevention and treatment of corticosteroid induced bone loss. *J Rheumatol* 2000; **27**: 2424–2431.

116. Saag GG, Emkey R, Schnitzer TJ *et al*. Alendronate for the prevention and treatment of glucocorticoid-induced osteoporosis. *New Engl J Med* 1998; **339**: 292–299.

117. Reid DM, Hughes RA, Laan RF *et al*. Efficacy and safety of daily risedronate in the treatment of corticosteroid-induced osteoporosis in men and women: a randomized trial. European Corticosteroid-Induced Osteoporosis Treatment Study. *J Bone Miner Res* 2000; **15**: 1006–1013.

118. Healey JH, Paget SA, Williams-Russo P *et al*. A randomized controlled trial of salmon calcitonin to prevent bone loss in corticosteroid-treated temporal arteritis and polymyalgia rheumatica. *Calcif Tiss Int* 1996; **58**: 73–80.

119. Sambrook P, Birmingham J, Kelly P *et al*. Prevention of corticosteroid osteoporosis. A comparison of calcium, calcitriol, and calcitonin. *New Engl J Med* 1993; **328**: 1747–1752.

120. Baillie SP, Davison CE, Johnson FJ, Francis RM. Pathogenesis of vertebral crush fractures in men. *Age Ageing* 1992; **21**: 139–141.

121. Francis RM. Male osteoporosis. *Rheumatology (Oxford)* 2000; **39**: 1055–1057.

122. Orwoll ES, Bevan L, Phipps KR. Determinants of bone mineral density in older men. *Osteoporosis Int* 2000; **11**: 815–821.

123. Khosla S, Melton LJ III, Riggs BL. Estrogens and bone health in men. *Calcif Tiss Int* 2001; **69**: 189–192.

124. Soroko SB, Barret-Connor E, Edelstein SL, Kritz-Silverstein D. Family history of osteoporosis and bone mineral density at the axial skeleton: the Rancho Bernardo study. *J Bone Miner Res* 1994; **9**: 761–769.

125. Kannus P, Palvanen M, Kaprio J *et al*. Genetic factors and osteoporotic fractures in elderly people: prospective 25 year follow up of a nationwide cohort of elderly Finnish twins. *Br Med J* 1999; **319**: 1334–1337.

126. Gennari L, Brandi ML. Genetics of male osteoporosis. *Calcif Tiss Int* 2001; **69**: 200–204.

127. Orwoll ES, Belknap JK, Klein RF. Gender specificity in the genetic determinants of peak bone mass. *J Bone Miner Res* 2001; **16**: 1962–1971.

128. Faulkner KG, Orwoll E. Implications in the use of T-scores for the diagnosis of osteoporosis in men. *J Clin Densitom* 2002; **5**: 87–93.

129. Anderson FH, Francis RM, Faulkner K. Androgen supplementation in eugonadal men with osteoporosis – effects of 6 months of treatment on bone mineral density and cardiovascular risk factors. *Bone* 1996; **18**: 171–177.

130. Orwoll E, Ettinger M, Weiss S *et al*. Alendronate for the treatment of osteoporosis in men. *New Engl J Med* **343**: 604–610.

131. Ringe JD, Dorst A, Kipshoven C *et al*. Avoidance of vertebral fractures in men with idiopathic osteoporosis by a three year therapy with calcium and low-dose intermittent monofluorophosphate. *Osteoporosis Int* 1998; **8**: 47–52.

132. Byers PH. Osteogenesis imperfecta: perspectives and opportunities. *Curr Opin Pediatr* 2000; **12**: 603–609.

133. Glorieux FH, Ward LM, Rauch F *et al*. Osteogenesis imperfecta type VI: a form of brittle bone disease with a mineralization defect. *J Bone Miner Res* 2002; **17**: 30–38.

134. Glorieux FH, Rauch F, Plotkin H *et al*. Type V osteogenesis imperfecta: a new form of brittle bone disease. *J Bone Miner Res* 2000; **15**: 1650–1658.

135. Boyde A, Travers R, Glorieux FH, Jones SJ. The mineralization density of iliac crest bone from children with osteogenesis imperfecta. *Calcif Tiss Int* 1999; **64**: 185–190.

136. Glorieux FH, Bishop NJ, Plotkin H *et al*. Cyclic administration of pamidronate in children with severe osteogenesis imperfecta. *New Engl J Med* 1998; **339**: 947–952.

137. Paterson CR, McAllion S, Stellman JL. Osteogenesis imperfecta after the menopause. *New Engl J Med* 1984; **310**: 1694–1696.

138. Lorenc RS. Idiopathic juvenile osteoporosis. *Calcif Tiss Int* 2002; **70**:395–397.

139. Shaw NJ, Boivin CM, Crabtree NJ. Intravenous pamidronate in juvenile osteoporosis. *Arch Dis Child* 2000; **83**: 143–145.

140. Smith R, Phillips AJ. Osteoporosis during pregnancy and its management. *Scand J Rheumatol Suppl* 1998; **107**: 66–67.

Appendix 1 – Drugs Used to Treat Osteoporosis

Drug	Trade name	Dose	Regimen	Comments	Most common side effects
Alendronate	Fosamax	10 mg	One tablet daily. Take on an empty stomach with a large glass of water, at least 1 hour before and 3 hours after food	Do not take with other medications. Use with caution in patients with gastro-oesophageal reflux disease. Contraindicated in patients with oesophageal stricture	Heartburn, dyspepsia, oesophageal ulceration
Alendronate	Fosamax	70 mg	One tablet weekly. Take on an empty stomach with a large glass of water at least 1 hour before and 3 hours after food	As above. Better tolerated than daily Alendronate	As above
Etidronate/calcium	Didronel PMO	400 mg etidronate/ 1000 mg calcium citrate	Take one etidronate tablet daily for 14 days on an empty stomach with a large glass of water, at least 1 hour before and 3 hours after food. Take one calcium tablet daily for 76 days. Resume etidronate and repeat on a cyclical basis	Do not take with other medications	

Drug	Trade name	Dose	Regimen	Comments	Most common side effects
Risedronate	Actonel	5 mg	One tablet daily. Take on an empty stomach with a large glass of water, at least 1 hour before and 3 hours after food	Do not take with other medications. Use with caution in patients with gastro-oesophageal reflux disease. Contraindicated in patients with oesophageal stricture	Headache
Risedronate	Actonel	35mg	One tablet weekly	As above	As above
Raloxifene	Evista	60 mg	One tablet daily with or without food	Increases risk of VTE. Reduces risk of breast cancer	Muscle cramps, hot flushes
Calcitonin (intranasal)	Miacalcin	200 IU	Take one puff intranasally each day		Rhinitis, epistaxis, headache
Calcitonin (injectable)	Calcynar	100 IU	One injection daily, subcutaneously	May have analgesic effect in acute vertebral fracture	Hot flushes, nausea, vomiting
Tibolone	Livial	2.5 mg	One tablet daily with or without food	Improves libido and helps menopausal vasomotor symptoms	Hirsutism
Parathyroid hormone	Forteo	20 mcg	One injection daily for 18–24 months	Indicated to increase bone mass in severe osteoporosis	Nausea, headache and hypercalcaemia

Drug	Trade name	Dose	Regimen	Comments	Most common side effects
Hormone replacement therapy	Various formulations	Various doses	Various regimes	Improves libido and helps menopausal vasomotor symptoms	Weight gain, fluid retention, breast tenderness, menstrual bleeding, increased risk of breast cancer and vascular disease with prolonged use
1,25-Dihydroxyvitamin D	Rocaltrol	250 mg daily	1–2 tablets daily	Monitor serum calcium and renal function during treatment	Hypercalcaemia
Calcium supplements	Various formulations	500–1000 mg	1–2 tablets daily	Indicated in patients with low dietary calcium; used as an adjunct to other agents in treatment of established osteoporosis	Gastrointestinal upset
Calcium and vitamin D supplements	Various formulations	500–1000 mg calcium; 400–800 IU cholecalciferol	1–2 tablets daily	Indicated in patients with low dietary calcium and vitamin D, and for the primary prevention of fractures in the elderly; used as an adjunct to other agents in treatment of established osteoporosis	Gastrointestinal upset

Appendix 2 – Useful Websites

Societies
American Society for Bone and Mineral Research
(http://www.asbmr.org)
European Calcified Tissues Society
(http://www.ectsoc.org/)
International Bone and Mineral Society
(http://www.ibmsonline.org/)
International Osteoporosis Foundation
(http://www.osteofound.org/)
National Osteoporosis Society (UK)
(http://www.nos.org.uk/)
National Osteoporosis Foundation (US)
(http://www.nof.org/)

Journals
Bone
(http://www.ibmsonline.org/bone/about.cfm)
Calcified Tissue International
(http://link.springer-ny.com/link/service/journals/
00223/index.htm)
Journal of Bone and Mineral Research
(http://www.jbmr-online.org/)
Osteoporosis International
(http://link.springer-ny.com/link/service/journals/
00198/index.htm)

Index

Note: As Osteoporosis is the major subject of the book, all
index entries refer to osteoporosis unless otherwise
indicated. Page numbers followed by 'f' indicate
figures; page numbers followed by 't' indicate tables.
HRT - hormone replacement therapy